'Dr Elliot Cohen draws on contempc
spiritual traditions, East and West, to
this way, we gain joy and wholeness.'

– **Edward Hoffman, Ph.D.,** *Au...*
to Add Joy to Your Life Every Day

'What a beautiful book!

Dr Cohen reminds us of a wisdom and a way of being which transcends and cuts through the malignant rush of modern living. Through unparalleled insights into Hinduism, Buddhism, Daoism and Judaism, we are invited to rediscover the "still, small voice of calm", often unheard but always present, if we have the presence of mind to listen. These are insights which are too often overlooked when considering why we struggle, in the way that we struggle and when we struggle.

An essential read for psychiatrists, psychologists and anyone wishing to understand more about Slow Living, this book is an absolute joy.'

– **Dr Anoop Mohan, MRCPsych,** *Consultant Psychiatrist*

'Eloquent and learned, *The Psychology of Slow Living* offers us multiple perspectives from worldwide wisdom traditions on how we might learn to live in time, live more meditatively, more sensually and more consciously. Along the way Elliot Cohen introduces helpful interconnections between diverse systems of thought – from Tibetan Buddhism and Daoism to the biophilia of Fromm and Wilson to his own reflections and experiences of the Jewish day of rest, and its deeper implications worked out in the kabbalah of the Zohar.

This is a book to savor and contemplate as it leads us to slow down and contemplate the world and our lives with greater care and love.'

– **Professor Rodger Kamenetz, PhD,** *Author of* The Jew in the Lotus
and The History of Last Night's Dream

'This book was a practical masterpiece, written in a clear, simple language, to inspire and invite the reader to cultivate a culture of slowing down – for one's life and wellbeing.

The author navigates admirably through the ancient wisdoms of Hinduism, Buddhism, Daoism and Judaism, explaining their interconnectedness.

Stillness is the gateway to serenity, clarity, harmony and authenticity. This is an outstanding explanation of the deep spiritual and psychological essence of slow living.'

– **Venerable Akurala Samitha,** *Head Monk at the Dhamma Nikethanaya Buddhist Academy*

THE PSYCHOLOGY OF SLOW LIVING

This fascinating book explores the concept of slow living, offering a philosophical and psychological exploration of the need for a slower pace of life. It advocates for reclaiming and rediscovering more natural and human ways of being.

In a digital age, which is dominated by an increasingly tyrannical trinity of speed, efficiency and productivity, the author challenges the pernicious ideal of instant gratification, perpetuated by modern consumer culture. This book examines alternative ways of being through re-examining the Wisdom Traditions of Hinduism, Buddhism, Daoism and Judaism through an ongoing and engaging dialogue with psychology and psychotherapy, including insights from environmental psychology, ecopsychology and cyberpsychology. The book argues against the trend for personal responsibility, adaptability and resilience, and the idea that stress is the 'new normal'. Instead, it proposes a radical shift in paradigm, promoting not for collectively rising up and overthrowing this system but for communally sitting down and reimagining.

The Psychology of Slow Living is a unique exploration of the benefits of the slow living movement and taps into contemporary debates around the way we should be living our lives, making it an ideal resource for students and academics in psychology, philosophy and the social sciences, as well as individuals interested in alternative lifestyles and spirituality.

Dr Elliot Cohen is a chartered psychologist and associate fellow of the British Psychological Society, senior lecturer in social psychology and interdisciplinary psychology at Leeds Beckett University, and the current Chair of the British Psychological Society's Transpersonal Psychology Section. He has over twenty years of experience in Hindu, Buddhist and Daoist contemplative traditions and is an authorised teacher of mindfulness meditation (Dhamma Nikethanaya Buddhist Academy). He has previously lectured in comparative religion at Manchester University and worked as a researcher for BBC Religion and Ethics.

THE PSYCHOLOGY OF SLOW LIVING

Rediscovering a Happier Pace of Life

Elliot Cohen

Routledge
Taylor & Francis Group
LONDON AND NEW YORK

Designed cover image: Getty Images via William Yu Photography

First published 2025
by Routledge
4 Park Square, Milton Park, Abingdon, Oxon OX14 4RN

and by Routledge
605 Third Avenue, New York, NY 10158

Routledge is an imprint of the Taylor & Francis Group, an informa business

British Library Cataloguing-in-Publication Data
A catalogue record for this book is available from the British Library

ISBN: 9781032370323 (hbk)
ISBN: 9781032362236 (pbk)
ISBN: 9781003334972 (ebk)

DOI: 10.4324/9781003334972

Typeset in Sabon LT Pro
by Apex CoVantage, LLC

CONTENTS

PREFACE – WHY SLOW LIVING?

Whenever I ask family, friends and colleagues how they are, I frequently receive an all too familiar reply 'Exhausted!'

The unrelenting and accelerating pace of modern life has run many of us ragged. It even seems that it is no longer deemed sufficient to run in order to keep up – our sugar-saturated, highly caffeinated energy drinks promise us wings with which to fly.

Quite clearly there are some areas of life where speed is of the essence – receiving the results of an important medical test or undergoing a life-saving operation may be two such relatable examples. But increasingly, we appear to be extending an unnatural and unsustainable sense of urgency into almost all areas of our lives, living too intensely in a constant state of emergency – hyperactive, hypercognitive and hypervigilant.

The ubiquitous 'burnout' described in clinical literature, often precipitated by rising rates of anxiety disorders and depressive episodes, points to a common but often unarticulated conclusion – we can't go on like this, something needs to change. Despite all our repeated emphasis on increasing and fortifying psychological resilience, the time has come when many more people are questioning, 'What are we doing wrong that requires us all to be so resilient so often?'

Rather than seeking a deeper, comprehensive answer, our shortcut culture typically tends to look for a quick fix, a life hack or mind hack that will lessen the symptoms whilst leaving the underlying causes largely unaddressed and consequently untreated.

A great many popular wellness trends, fads and fashions all appear to share many of the same themes and features. We may be encouraged to live more purposefully through the Japanese method of *Ikigai*, cultivate physical and psychological flexibility through the practice of Yoga, or to take more mindful moments during our day, all with the intention of discovering a more healthy, harmonious and happier way of life.

Of all these trends, one of the most popular and persistent has been mindfulness. Mindfulness occupies a privileged position within the burgeoning well-being industry, supported by a sturdy evidence base of peer-reviewed research – spawning numerous Mindfulness-Based Interventions, accredited degree and diploma programmes, week-long and weekend retreats, and a multitude of mobile phone apps. The 'Mindfulness Revolution' appeared to be the promised panacea to the particular ills of our age. Critics soon emerged who challenged the unrealistic claims of a universal remedy, whilst also decrying the many ways mindfulness was being misappropriated, commodified and monetised. Mindfulness can all too easily become just another stress-relief technique rather than the profound, spiritually transformative practice Buddhists understand it to be.

What is sorely needed is a more fundamental shift in our thinking and lifestyles.

I have found that *Slow Living* encompasses all the aforementioned themes and features whilst having the added benefit of emphasising that this practice constitutes a whole *way of life* – it also crucially recognises that our *way* of life is largely determined by our *pace* of life. But slow living is challenging.

The challenge becomes most evident when the same restless mindset that lies at the root of so much of our suffering is employed to seek a solution. We may consequently find ourselves in the paradoxical predicament of being in a hurry to slow down. We may race to embrace the principles and employ practices of slow living with only a surface understanding of this holistic endeavour.

This book strives to provide the much-needed psychological, philosophical and spiritual foundations of Slow Living, in order to inform, support and maintain such a shift in thinking and lifestyle.

I present Slow Living as a corrective lens intended to counter a myopic vision of a world habitually distorted by speed and greed. Its seven chapters offer different world views inspired by varied wisdom traditions, coupled with psychological insights, presenting meaningful, alternative ways of seeing and being.

ACKNOWLEDGEMENTS

For Zhilu, Natan and Ezra and the Cohen Family – Henry and Margaret, Dan and Elayna.

With special thanks to Leeds Beckett University's (LBU) Centre for Applied Social Research (CEASR), Professor Livia Kohn, Professor Michael Saso, Professor Les Lancaster, Professor Karl Spracklen, Professor Daniel Matt, Professor Bryan Van Norden, Professor Paul Swanson, Professor David Chai, Lama Jampa Thaye, Dr Debashish Banerji, Dr Paul Taberham, Dr Conrad Russell, Dr Valerie Roebuck, Dr Jeffrey Kotyk, Dr Nisha Gupta, Rabbi Dr Cody Bahir, Rabbi Danny Bergson, Rev. Dr Alasdair Gordon-Finlayson, Rev. Jikai Dehn, Dr Unjyn Park, Dr Jenni Myers, Dr Winnie Bedigen, Stephen Sayers, Harkiran Sahota, Richard Cohen, Yuka Hirano, Masaya Okamoto, Lowell Cook, Ian Baker, Cittaslow, Menorah Synagogue, The British Daoist Association, The Samatha Trust, Tendai Buddhism UK, The BPS Transpersonal Psychology Section, and to all my current and past students at LBU's Social Psychology BA(Hons) and Interdisciplinary Psychology MA.

1

SLOW AND FAST LIVING

This book was originally inspired by a simple motorway sign that read 'Speed Kills, Slow Down'.

This sign, with its stark and sobering message, serves to remind us just how quickly we can become accustomed and desensitised to speed and its inherent dangers. Cocooned in the seemingly safe metal casing of our cars, we collectively race towards our respective destinations. The race however is seldom smooth or without delays. The sheer volume of traffic constantly competing for space leads paradoxically to increasing congestion and obstructions. In our determined quest to save time, we lose time, and in seeking to go faster, we seem to go ever slower.

Such everyday experiences only serve to further amplify our associations of slowness with irritation, inconvenience and stress, and by marked contrast we come to associate speed with the freedom of the much mythologised but seldom realised open road.

The sheer number of cars on the road requires that motorways themselves be in an almost constant state of maintenance and repair, in addition to the perpetual projects of expansion and extension – all leading to yet further delay and inconvenience.

The familiar experience of frustration whilst being stationary on a motorway is ubiquitous and yet we seldom see or recognise our personal responsibility. Environmentalists seek to remind and reproach us with slogans, such as 'You are not stuck in traffic – you ARE traffic!' Similarly, I recall experiencing a Zen-like flash of insight when a particularly exacerbated London Cabbie exclaimed, as we crawled along Fleet Street, 'No one drives in London anymore, there's too much traffic!'

DOI: 10.4324/9781003334972-1

Feeling increasingly trapped, like rats in a cage, or reluctant competitors in the great 'rat race', one might recall the research of John Calhoun's (1970) arguably cruel and curiously named rat and mouse 'Utopia' experiments. Over several decades, Calhoun studied overcrowding in rodent populations and repeatedly observed a disturbing and predictable period of 'behavioural sink'. This term conveyed a marked physical, behavioural and psychological deterioration. Increasing competition and the resultant stress led to violence – torn ears, chewed tails, even incidences of cannibalism, mothers abandoning their young, and some traumatised rodents withdrawing completely into self-centred isolation. Comparative Psychologists and Environmental Psychologists still look to this study as a dire warning for what could happen to humanity were our numbers to increase beyond our capacity to adequately care for or even about one another.

In the daily grind of gridlocked traffic, amidst choking fumes, we too may observe or experience our very own 'behavioural sink', now described with a more familiar term – 'road rage'. This term evokes all too familiar scenes or 'symptoms' of formerly calm and kind individuals suddenly screaming profanities whilst aggressively gesticulating at complete strangers, angrily sounding horns, intimidatingly tailing vehicles, or recklessly overtaking or undertaking at dangerous speeds, leading to the potentially fatal crash that all too frequently follows.

Upon further reflection, one can begin to understand how the very existence of cars and motorways, and the industrial revolutions that preceded them, exemplifies our culture's single-minded pursuit, fetishisation and commercialisation of speed – our *velocentricity.*

The first industrial revolution of the nineteenth century had been the age of steam and locomotion, signalling the rapid rise of railways, factories and the origins of urbanisation. This was also the age of empire and innovation, colonialism and oppression, with a renewed emphasis on and passion for *speed, efficiency and productivity* – the increasingly tyrannical trinity of modernity.

Minds were rapidly transforming alongside landscapes, as Romantic poets such as Blake deeply lamented the loss of the English countryside – the familiar, traditional, pastoral scenes and their sudden replacement with black, belching chimneys. In his iconic poem 'And Did Those Feet in Ancient Time', Blake nostalgically recalls the former Arcadian allure of 'England's mountains green', contrasted with the new 'dark satanic mills' (Blake 1893, p. 207). The poetic and theological themes of a paradise lost were to become a frequent staple in the Romantic poetry of the era, and still persist into the twenty-first century. Over a century later, the poem was to become a very popular Anglican hymn and is still frequently sung to express all that is, or was, quintessentially English – while the uplifting melody suggests hope, the lyrics openly mourn what has been destroyed and pines for a new Jerusalem.

The velocentric mindset was to become ever more vigorous and entrenched when Henry Ford's production lines revolutionised the automotive industry at the beginning of the twentieth century, initiating the second industrial revolution. The time taken to manufacture Ford cars, specifically the Model T chassis, reduced significantly – beginning as a process taking over twelve hours, reducing to six hours, until they historically achieved an hour and a half assembly time (Halberstam 2003, p. 66).

Fordism heralded a new age of increasingly mechanised, rapid, mass production and consequently mass consumption, emphasising and prioritising economic growth and social order. Ford's particular fixation with order was not limited to the factory but extended into all areas of public life with a fascistic intensity. The Henry Ford Sociological Department and English School could closely monitor and regulate the private lives of factory workers, with a notable preoccupation with conformity and homogeneity. The graduation ceremony for the English School was particularly revealing:

> students were transformed into Americans. During the ceremony speakers gave rousing patriotic speeches and factory bands played marches and patriotic songs. The highlight of the event would be the transformation of immigrants into Americans. Students dressed in costumes reminiscent of their native homes stepped into a massive stage-prop cauldron that had a banner across the front identifying it as the AMERICAN MELTING POT. Seconds later, after a quick change out of sight of the audience, students emerged wearing 'American' suits and hats, waving American flags, having undergone a spiritual smelting process where the impurities of foreignness were burnt off as slag to be tossed away leaving a new 100% American.
>
> *(The Henry Ford 2022)*

Ford required his workers to conform to his particular expectations and standardised specifications for what constituted an American, in a similar manner to the way he demanded uniformity in his vehicles. Ford's preference for marching music and patriotic songs may also be significant; encouraging a more mechanised, lockstep way of moving, thinking and feeling. Ford was particularly disturbed and incensed by the increasing popularity of Jazz in his day – condemning the free-flowing, loose, spontaneous, occasionally chaotic rhythms and melodies as 'Jewish Jazz – Moron Music' (Ford 1921).

Improvisation is the beating heart of Jazz, but improvisation is diametrically opposed to automation; Jazz plays with order, acoustically subverting, audibly parodying it, which is likely one of the key reasons the genre was banned by authoritarian regimes, including Nazi Germany and the Soviet Union. Jazz as an emerging musical genre represented a very different kind of melting pot, frequently featuring Jewish and Black musicians, encouraging varied forms of interracial mixing which horrified Ford. It is ironic that one of Ford's favourite images of America as 'The Melting Pot' was itself originally popularised by the Jewish playwright Israel Zangwill.

Despite Ford's well-documented, openly fascist sympathies and vocal antisemitic sentiments, the Ford car became and remains an iconic symbol of American ingenuity, prosperity and modernist progress. Car ownership was itself to become emblematic of success, an integral part of achieving the American dream – driving towards Life, Liberty and the Pursuit of Happiness. Similarly, in 1937, Adolf Hitler would promote the *Volkswagen*, literally the 'People's Car', as an integral part of his vision for a prosperous and industrious Germany; a new potent, mobile symbol of and centrepiece for the Third Reich. Patriotic consumers, American or German, could now increasingly afford to buy their way into being significant players in these new national narratives of modernity and progress.

The subsequent emergence of a consumer culture further reified formerly lifeless objects that had previously served practical needs, to tantalising, highly desired objects, as Marx had first described in *Das Kapital* in 1867, when Capitalism was still in its relative infancy:

> A commodity appears at first sight an extremely obvious, trivial thing. But its analysis brings out that it is a very strange thing, abounding in metaphysical subtleties and theological niceties.
>
> *(Marx 1990, p. 163)*

The car as a commodity was no mere, simple assemblage of mechanical parts but had come to increasingly symbolise innovation, individualism and freedom itself. Semiotic analyses of car advertisements, particularly evident from the 1950s onwards, reveal that the car is not only a prized or desired possession but is increasingly understood and related to as a reflection and extension of the owner (Gordon and Suzuki 1991); the sports car soon comes to signify virility and youth, freedom and ambition, while contrastingly, the family car signifies steadiness, safety and reliability. In subtle yet progressively tangible ways, we begin to become ever more defined and even possessed by our possessions. Humanistic Psychoanalyst Erich Fromm was particularly critical of the types of 'nonfunctional (irrational) consumption' (Fromm 2001, p. 115) he saw displayed in car ownership:

> One would need to write a book in order to give a full description of the irrational and pathogenic function of the type of consumption that the private automobile represents.
>
> *(Ibid.)*

In popular culture, the car and the open highway came to represent personal choice, new freedoms, horizons and opportunities. Almost every road movie involves an obligatory voyage of discovery and personal growth. Popular songs such as Tracy Chapman's 'Fast Car' contain all those aforementioned attributes, including the seductive promises of belonging and being someone (Chapman 1988).

Twenty-first-century attitudes towards the car are far more ambivalent. Contemporary consumers increasingly reflect on the environmental costs of our convenience. The ever-present and rising spectre of climate catastrophe, with accompanying, familiar green rhetoric relating to 'carbon footprints' and 'sustainability', is gradually transforming our perception of the car – revealing evermore inconvenient truths about this convenient form of transport, as we recognise its significant role in exacerbating both local levels of pollution and the global climate emergency.

Increasingly, we are being encouraged by both national and local governments, health authorities and Green campaigners to walk or to bike as both a healthy and environmentally friendly alternative to driving. This is not such a recent innovation however – earlier alternative forms of vélocentrism may be encountered in countercultural movements that promoted 'vélorutionary perspectives' (Ryle and Soper 2013, p. 101).

This vélorutionary perspective, inspired by bicycle activists of Amsterdam and Montreal during the 1960s and 1970s, sees in the bike an enduring symbol for a more humanised pace and way of life. The bicycle's speed is determined by one's intention, effort and endurance through pedalling, as opposed to the comparatively undemanding press of a car's accelerator pedal. In the car, one typically, impersonally speeds through spaces and places in an almost unconscious, automatised, indiscriminate manner, until one arrives at one's destination, often remembering little of the journey – whereas walking and biking allow for a far more aesthetically immersive, experientially rich, and memorable journey.

For vélorutionaries, the car was seen as a signifier of authoritarianism and the dehumanising cult of speed; exemplified earlier in Henry Ford's fascist leanings. This is not to say that the bike itself is entirely immune from pervasive velocentric tendencies, as it too can easily become a dehumanising and competitive tool intended for the 'smashing' of world records on roads and in purpose-built velodromes, or else motorised:

> Italian futurism offers an historical example of the link between speed-worship and fascism (Marinetti 1909; cf. Virilio 1977, 2003). When the bike is fetishized as a speed-machine, cycling becomes not the antithesis but the very sign of turbo-culture's conquest of mind and body: flesh is imagined as steel, rather than vice versa.
>
> *(Ryle and Soper 2013, pp. 103–104)*

The reference to the Italian artist Marinetti (1909) is of particular significance as his publication 'The Founding and Manifesto of Futurism' called for a cultural revolution where tradition was to be superseded and replaced with an unbridled celebration of speed and power as described in the fourth clause of the manifesto:

> We declare that the splendor of the world has been enriched by a new beauty: the beauty of speed. A racing automobile with its bonnet adorned with great tubes like serpents with explosive breath . . . a roaring motor car which seems to run on machine-gun fire, is more beautiful than the Victory of Samothrace.
>
> *(Marinetti 1909)*

This new beauty, the aesthetics of acceleration, appeared to pave the way for a more violent and mechanistic mankind, as clause nine states:

> We will glorify war – the world's only hygiene – militarism, patriotism, the destructive gesture of freedom-bringers, beautiful ideas worth dying for.
>
> *(Ibid.)*

In Marinetti-inspired, Italian Futurist art, such as Fortunato Depero's paintings 'Patriotic Storm Marinetti' (referred to as a psychological portrait) or 'The Motorcyclist', one can vividly encounter the human form reimagined – menacingly morphing into sharper, more angular, steel-like forms. Italian futurism and fascism seemed destined to align as Marinetti forged close ties with Benito Mussolini in 1919, appearing at political rallies together, simultaneously promoting the futurist and fascist cause. For Marinetti, Mussolini seemingly embodied the strength, speed and militarism futurism strived for – a rapidly re-envisioned Italy.

This intimate relationship between speed and war was further explored in French historian and philosopher, Paul Virilio's (2007) 'Speed and Politics', where he critically examined the previous industrial revolutions, political systems and global conflicts in relation to what he terms 'dromology'. The etymological roots of dromology are found in the Greek term δρόμος *drómos*, referring to racing or running. Virilio's assessment is quite striking as he reflects on the violence of speed and the accelerating, exhausting pace of technology; explicitly linking the pace of the arms race with the progression of history.

> In fact, there was no 'industrial revolution,' but only a 'dromocratic revolution;' there is no democracy, only dromocracy; there is no strategy, only dromology.
>
> *(Virilio 2007, p. 69)*

The industrial revolutions continue apace, each promising greater speed, convenience and connectivity, but delivering just as much anxiety, novel obstacles and alienation.

The 1980s saw the dawning of the Digital Age, a third industrial revolution catalysed by the invention of the internet – a new cyber-Jerusalem, with virtual mountains and pastures to explore. Exchanging the freedom of the highway for driving or surfing on the information superhighway.

Our current fourth industrial age (4.0), swiftly transforming into a fifth industrial age (5.0), appears to have extended the domain of the digital into almost all areas of daily life, with the pervasive algorithms that dictate, shape or determine our online experience, attitudes and behaviours; coupled with the rapid rise of generative Artificial Intelligence with its potentially apocalyptic repercussions. But our insatiable appetite for speed appears unabated.

From Fast Cars to Fast Food

> Tell me what you eat and I will tell you who you are.
>
> (Anthelme Brillat-Savarin quoted in Gabaccia 2009, p. 225)

This quote from a noted nineteenth-century French jurist and gourmet is the most likely source for the popular English adage 'you are what you eat'. The study of the social psychology of food (Connor and Armitage 2002) reminds us that it is not simply a matter of *what* we eat, but also why, where and with whom we eat. Food and our relationship to it is no simple matter of mere sustenance. Food may constitute a core component of one's social and cultural identity, being at the centre of most family and communal gatherings. Additionally, it is often used to provide emotional comfort or support during times of stress. Subsequently, the shadow aspect of food, its abuse, is encountered in the rising prevalence and variety of eating disorders; with clinical literature concerning eating disorders often centring around the two extremes of obesity and anorexia. The obesity epidemic in particular, identified by the World Health Organisation, is frequently singled out as an issue for global concern, and one that has only been further exacerbated by the recent global pandemic, where so many stayed indoors and increasingly *binged* on both food and entertainment streaming services, as there seemed so little else to do – excess quickly became the norm.

If Futurism reflected the mid-twentieth century's love of speed and power, then perhaps the twenty-first century may be characterised by the artistic movement of Excessivism:

> Capitalism has created a new social paradigm in which consumption is no longer related to basic need satisfaction, but rather to the creation and production of a sense of self based solely on the excessive and incessant consumption of material goods.
>
> *(Marta Nelson 2022)*

The Excessivism movement seeks to explore and creatively critique the complex relationships between consumer culture and identity – reflecting our 'cultures of excess' (Slosar 2009). One commonly identified culprit is the fast food industry.

The increasing prevalence and popularity of fast food outlets in the US, beginning in the 1950s, convincingly demonstrated how our enduring appetite for speed had moved beyond the aesthetic into the dietetic. Seemingly every element of 'fast food' beginning at production and ending in consumption serves to further embed and embody the velocentric mindset, leading to a velocentric menu.

In many significant ways, McDonaldism appears as the natural successor to Fordism, with its emphases on speed, productivity, efficiency and consistency. The instantly recognisable golden arches of the McDonald's corporation promise a uniformity of product, swift service and eating experience, irrespective of one's geographical location – from London to Beijing, this is one familiar way that the process of globalisation leads to homogenisation.

When American Sociologist George Ritzer (2015) writes about the process of 'McDonaldisation', he explicitly makes the comparison between McDonaldism and Fordism. McDonaldisation as a process is described as having four main characteristics or emphases – efficiency, calculability, predictability and control through technology.

Once again, there are some notable overlaps with the Italian Futurists who also emphasised in their 1932 *La Cucina Futurista* – The Futurist Cookbook, the importance of food arriving swiftly with a striking appearance, often being deemed more important than the taste – in fact, some of the food to be presented was intended for display purposes only. One is perhaps reminded of the familiar contrast between the almost magical, glossy, mouth-watering depictions of the food on the menus of fast food outlets, compared with the disappointing, lacklustre lunch that arrives at one's table somewhat compressed and somehow disenchanted.

For futurists, much was also made of the utilisation of technology in the process of food production, involving 'a battery of scientific instruments in the kitchen' (Marinetti 2014, p. 30) including smell-enhancing ozonisers, ultraviolet lamps to activate vitamins and chemical analysers to determine the acidity or alkalinity of the sauces. In regard to nutrition, one also encounters an unsettling vision of a new nationalist food culture:

> We invite chemistry immediately to take on the task of providing the body with its necessary calories through equivalent nutrients provided free by the State, in powder and pills, albumoid compounds, synthetic fats and vitamins.
>
> *(Ibid., p. 30)*

Their vision represented an all-out assault on long-established Italian culinary tastes and traditions, to the extent that they even proposed pasta be entirely removed from the menu! The Futurists claimed that the consumption of pasta led to a slower, bloated, less virile and more lethargic nation; as for advocates of this national dish, the 'defenders of pastasciutta', they denounced:

> They do not have the spiritual lucidity of the laboratory. They forget the lofty dynamic obligations of the race and the searing speed and most violent contradictory forces that constitute the agonizing rush of modern life.
> *(Ibid., p. 31)*

This was an explicit effort to change and conform hearts and minds through diet – fast food for a faster, fascistic nation.

Perhaps it is appropriate therefore that a rising resistance to both the futurist agenda and fast food also began in Italy in the 1980s.

Slow Food and Slow Culture

Futurism and Fast Food find their antithesis in the Slow Food movement, founded by Carlo Petrini.

Petrini, who had his political roots firmly planted in the Italian Left, founded the 'Slow Food' movement in Italy in 1989, but his activism had begun three years earlier in 1986 under the more politically-charged name Arcigola. The acronym ARCI stood for *Associazione Ricreativa dei Comunisti Italiani* – the Recreational Association of Italian Communists, with the suffix *gola* referring to throat, indicating eating or gluttony.

Their early protests took place in direct opposition to the McDonalds Corporation's efforts to open a restaurant in Rome's Piazza di Spagna, one of Italy's most iconic landmarks located in the heart of the capital. It is also significant that one of the more publicised forms of protest involved protestors handing out bowls of penne pasta that would then be slowly consumed. The choice of pasta appears highly symbolic both as a reclamation of traditional Italian food culture and as a tangible, edible way to resist what they saw as a hegemonic drive towards homogenisation and globalisation by celebrating and emphasising the distinctiveness, variety and authenticity of the local cuisine. The protests were however ultimately unsuccessful and today the McDonald's restaurant at the Piazza di Spagna is just one of the fifty-four located in Rome alone. Despite this, the Slow Food movement has, over the last forty years, been successfully, steadily growing far beyond its hometown, the Italian town of Bra, currently having supporters and activists in over one hundred and sixty countries.

Despite the name 'Slow Food', the scope of the movement is much broader and multifaceted. Their 1989 'Official Manifesto for the International Movement for the Defence of and the Right to Pleasure' begins:

> Our century, which began and has developed under the insignia of industrialisation, first invented the machine and then took it as its like model.
>
> We are enslaved by speed and have all succumbed to the same insidious virus: *Fast Life*, which disrupts our habits, pervades the privacy of our homes and forces us to eat *Fast Foods*.
>
> *(quoted in Parkins and Craig 2006, p. 141)*

Slow Food represents a grassroots resistance to and a quest for an alternative to the societal adoration of speed. The devotees of Dromology seek convenience, comfort and instant gratification – leading to the emergence of our contemporary click-and-collect culture, running alongside our communications revolution and the ubiquity of instant messaging.

From a psychoanalytic perspective, we may understand the demand for instant gratification as being related to what Freud termed the 'pleasure principle' (Laplanche and Pontalis 2004, p. 323). From the earliest moments of our awareness, we seek pleasure and the avoidance of unpleasure – the textbook example being a newborn infant experiencing the discomfort, or existential terror, of hunger and consequently screaming for their mother's milk. While this behaviour is accepted in infancy, it is increasingly frowned upon as we develop into early childhood. It is worth considering how much of our childhood was taken up with learning how to be patient, not to push or push in, to share and to wait for one's turn.

What we term adulthood is largely the end process of a lengthy period of socialisation during which we have learned to delay gratification in a more mature recognition of the existence and needs of others. The presence (real or imagined), needs and expectations of others, coupled with the apparent fact that we simply cannot have whatever we want whenever we want, should lead to a recognition of the 'reality principle' (Ibid., pp. 379–382). However, both the reality and principles that characterised Freud's day have arguably transformed beyond recognition, as our digital age appears to allow for almost every desire to be realised with a mere click on an icon – whatever the nature of the craving, as the popular saying goes 'there's an app for that'. How does the reality principle fare in the face of a novel virtual reality principle? Do those once fundamental and formative lessons of childhood still hold currency in an age where we are encouraged to expect ever more ever faster?

As with fast food, we may speedily receive the meal we desire, but does it do us any good nutritionally, psychologically or even spiritually? In light of current debates concerning both processed and ultra-processed food, one might reasonably ask whether it is still food at all. One might then conclude that our digitally enabled consumer culture is leading not towards any meaningful civilisational progress but in fact constituting a rapid atavistic regression, potentially culminating in our own extinction.

In E. M. Forster's dystopian science fiction, a short story first published in 1909 titled 'The Machine Stops' (Forster 2012), he eerily envisages, perhaps prophetically glimpses, a living death, a stagnating subterranean-dwelling humanity, entirely dependent on an all-powerful, global machine for all their needs. It is also significant that humanity is portrayed as being utterly alienated and cut off from the natural world with its rhythms and patterns of seasons and alternating periods of light and darkness, which are now all artificially replaced and regulated by the machine. The inhabitants of this world want for nothing and subsequently become as nothing.

Again, we might return to Psychoanalysis to consider the relationship between the pleasure principle and what Freud termed the Nirvana Principle (Laplanche and Pontalis 2004, pp. 272–273). In contrast to a more traditional Buddhist understanding of the term which connotes spiritual awakening and liberation, Freud links the Nirvana Principle to a later construct, which he termed the Death Drive. In opposition to the life-affirming and enhancing, nurturing and preserving force of *Eros*, Freud identifies the self-destructive drive of *Thanatos*, which includes the unconscious yearning to no longer exist. When one considers *Eros* and *Thanatos* in the twenty-first century, one can see how they relate to and reinforce one another – how our desire for comfort and convenience, for pleasure and the avoidance of unpleasure, has spawned the very lifestyles and industries that now threaten to disrupt and destroy our ecosystems and virtually end life as we know it.

We continuously, compulsively consume to excess with the fantasy that we might reach some sublime state of satiation, an idealised state of inertia where we too no longer need or desire anything at all. In this scenario, both desire and the existence predicated upon it appear utterly exhausted – yet we know that the nature of desire remains stubbornly insatiable, ever-evolving and adapting into more nuanced and subtler forms. Freud's 'Nirvana' is the pessimistic, nihilistic nirvana as understood by the philosopher Schopenhauer, not the joyful transcendence alluded to in the Buddhist scriptures, or the blissful union with the Divine described in the Hindu Scriptures as *Moksha*.

Despite Freud's study being filled with religious iconography and artefacts from around the world, his attitude towards religion appears consistently dismissive and reductive. For Freud, religion is frequently explained away as a regressive, infantile need for parental approval and protection, often taking the form of an externalised father figure, with mystical union being relegated to an unconscious longing to return to the blissful unawareness, pre-existence of the womb. When Freud's close friend, the French poet and novelist Romain Rolland ecstatically enthused about his study of Hindu spirituality, specifically the study of *Vedanta*, and wrote to Freud of a consciousness-transforming 'oceanic feeling', Freud replies rather matter-of-factly – 'I cannot discover this "oceanic" feeling in myself' (Freud quoted in Ackerman 2017, p. 19).

While Freud manifestly appears to reject religion, he still nevertheless clearly recognises the power and pull of its scriptural decrees and the appeal of its prophetic poetry as well as the abiding, semiotically-charged nature of its iconographies. Religion presents a great many ways to manage the onslaughts of the unconscious and the relentless demands of our desires, typically elevating various forms of repression, sublimation and expressions of renunciation, promoting the abandonment of the material in pursuit of the spiritual as exemplified in the many monastic and contemplative disciplines of both the East and the West. In addition to the various Buddhist statues, Daoist immortals and Hindu Deities that adorned Freud's study, he had also kept the Freud family bible in Hebrew, lovingly rebound and inscribed by his father Jacob Freud.

Freud's famous break with his former protégé, Carl Jung, was largely based on the latter's enthusiastic embracing and pursuit of spiritual experience and meaning in all their various forms. For Jung, the only authentic way to escape our various complexes, compulsions and addictions was to have a personal, transformative religious experience. Jung would assert, and many Transpersonal Psychologists would assent, that in order to effectively escape the hedonic treadmill, to transform and transcend our velocentric mindset, would necessarily require some form or degree of spiritual realisation, transformation or awakening. One notable outgrowth of the slow food movement has been the Cittaslow movement (*cittá* being the Italian word for city), which has, since its founding in 1999, called for a more collective awakening.

In the Cittaslow Manifesto (2023), the language seems to emulate a liturgical tone, recollecting the familiar scriptural form of the first verse of Genesis. On the Cittaslow website, one may even purchase this manifesto in the form of a 'precious parchment' (Ibid.):

> In the beginning man fed himself. He then sought shelter and protection: homes, villages, towns were founded. Finally, the time of the machines came with their increasingly hectic, frenetic rhythms of life. Today, man dreams of liberation from the many anxieties that his own progress has created.
>
> *(Ibid.)*

In addition to their parchment, the Cittaslow movement also has a unifying icon, the unassuming garden snail:

> 'A small, cosmopolitan and prudent' creature and an 'amulet against speed'.
>
> *(Kummer 2002 quoted in Parkins and Craig 2006, p. 19)*

The snail appears an obvious choice to signify slowness or slowing down. However, in relation to 'slow food', the snail may well appear as a counter-intuitive choice for a logo or amulet, considering that it is the bane of so many allotment keepers; greedily consuming all greenery. But the snail's symbolism is far richer and deeper than the mere surface appearance. If we engage in some Jungian *amplification*, we might deepen our appreciation for and transform our perception of this common 'garden pest'.

One of the most striking symbolic elements of the snail, quite prominent in the slow living logo, is the spiral shell. The spiral is a primordial and perennial form, a Klüverian form constant, found all around the world; frequently encountered in prehistoric petroglyphs, Shamanic art and religious iconography. The spiral is a multi-layered, labyrinthine symbol of journeying and of returning, of psychological and spiritual transformation.

In Buddhist iconography, one may notice a distinctive spiral pattern located in the region of the Buddha's 'third eye', which is more correctly a stylised tuft of light-emitting white hair called the *urna*, one of the traditional thirty-two marks of a great being. Indeed, all the Buddha's short shorn ringlets of hair quite often resemble small snail shells – there is even a popular oral tradition amongst Chinese Buddhists that pious, self-sacrificing snails would keep the Buddha's head cool during long periods of sitting meditation under the relentlessly hot Indian summer sun.

In early Christian symbolism also, the snail is associated with death and resurrection – this is in accordance with the medieval belief that the snail lived underground, within its shell – seemingly dead and inert, until it once again miraculously emerged – resurrecting and resurfacing with the warmer weather (Werness 2006, p. 376).

In the Cittaslow logo, one first sees the familiar snail and the spiral, but if one looks closer one can also see upon the snail's shell, resting upon it, there is the outline of a cityscape – reminding us that what started with simple slow food in more rural and pastoral settings is necessarily extending into our urban environments – leading to the creation of 'towns where living is good'. One such town is the UK town of Ludlow, located in the county of Shropshire.

The Pace of Place – Reflections in a Slow City

As I walked from my hotel, down Fishmore Road, towards the centre of Ludlow, I noticed a road sign, partially peppered with lichen, that fittingly read:

> Speed Limit Ahead. REDUCE SPEED NOW

Echoing the poet Blake, my souvenir guidebook informed me:

> Shropshire is a green and pleasant county with a wealth of timber-framed buildings, grand sandstone churches, ruined abbeys and country houses. Yet surprisingly this still largely rural county can justly claim to be the birthplace of the Industrial Revolution.
>
> *(Ruler 2010, p. 4)*

Both the Northerner and Mancunian in me took umbrage at this claim, as I knew Manchester to have been the first industrial city, Robert Stephenson's iconic steam engine 'The Rocket' had been built to run on the Liverpool and Manchester trainline in 1829, and I'd even taken my children to view it while it was on display at Manchester's Museum of Science and Industry. But now, I was being presented with a whole century earlier date of 1709, when Abraham Darby I, a Quaker and ironmaster, innovated using coke to smelt iron, which eventually led to the construction of the iron arch at Ironbridge Gorge in 1777. Despite this relatively brief industrial past, Shropshire had long since returned to its rural roots, and Ludlow had become a picture-perfect, idyllic English town. One resident proudly told me that their town was often voted to be one of the most beautiful places to live in Shropshire and the UK, and that this is the town many Londoners looking to 'downshift' flock to following their retirement from the rat race.

In 2003, Ludlow became the UK's first official slow town and member of the Cittaslow movement. In doing so, it sought to embody the Cittaslow vision of being a town that was

> animated by people 'curious about time reclaimed', rich in squares, theatres, workshops, cafes, restaurants, spiritual places, unspoilt landscapes and fascinating craftsmen, where we still appreciate the slow, benevolent succession of the seasons, with their rhythm of authentic products, respecting fine flavours and health, the spontaneity of their rituals, the fascination of living traditions. This is the joy of a slow, quiet, reflective way of life.
>
> *(Cittaslow Manifesto 2023)*

The Norman era castle, the bustling town market, the Tudor-style exteriors and Georgian brickwork all imbue the town with an instant imageability and sense of historicity. This is a perfect place to *dérive* or drift in the manner described by Psychogeographers – to consciously wander, allowing ample time to wonder, with an awakened appreciation for all the sights, sounds, scents and sensations that one might encounter. Ludlow is far from being another nondescript, standardised *space*, it is very much a humanised, personalised *place* (Benson 2001, p. 6). A fitting home for the Academy of Urbanism, as the town exemplifies placemaking, cultivating a strong, coherent place identity and topophilia (Tuan 1990).

If I appear to wax lyrical about Ludlow, it's because I was initially quite overcome by the tangible sense of serenity and calm compared to my hometown of Manchester. Perhaps it's only when we allow ourselves to take the time to slow down that we realise how fast we have been going and how much we have been carrying.

The terms allostatic load and overload are often used when discussing the cumulative psychological and physical toll of stress on the human body and mind (Schulkin 2004); its effects can be subtle and insidious – just as the joints and muscle pain is frequently felt most acutely the day following a marathon and not immediately after. Individually and collectively, we are typically encouraged and praised for both our ability and willingness to adapt to stressful conditions – in the well-being industry, one of the more popular buzzwords is that of 'resilience'. Even formerly spiritual practices such as mindfulness meditation, which has its original Buddhist roots in a more radical renunciation of worldly life and concerns, have been reimagined and repurposed within a more neoliberal ideology and agenda to enhance workers' resilience, increase efficiency and productivity, leading to what Ron Purser has termed 'McMindfulness' (Purser 2019). It is perhaps little wonder, as the entire world's economic models and priorities rest almost exclusively on productivity and consumption, myopically measuring a nation's success and standing according to Gross Domestic Product (GDP) – where market value often eclipses any competing human values or environmental concerns. The resultant obsession with quantification and metrics further fuels our cultures of excess, where we are led to believe we need ever more things even faster.

Remembering How to Slow Down

On March 23, 2020, the United Kingdom had its first national lockdown due to the global pandemic. The daily message was to 'Stay Home, Protect the NHS, Save Lives'. The whole country appeared to have stopped; only designated 'key workers' continued to work as millions more were furloughed. In addition to the daily statistics on the rising death rates, governments and economists noted with increasing alarm the declining rates of GDP worldwide.

Large segments of the British public, particularly the middle classes, collectively threw themselves into hobbies and activities. For several months, the imposed quarantine made people increasingly dependent on technology as part of a so-called 'new normal' – far from the machine stopping, this is arguably when the digital regime swiftly came to dominate our daily lives.

Social networking sites became saturated with shared posts, tweets and status updates of new budding bakers and gardeners. The lockdown was frequently presented as a great 'reset', a unique opportunity to 'downshift', to slow down and take account of one's life, questioning one's meaning, purpose and priorities. But for a great many it was a time of intense anxiety coupled with economic uncertainty – the psychological consequences of the lockdowns are still being assessed and addressed, including a resultant global mental health pandemic of stress and depression (WHO 2022).

In our habitual haste, so many simply could not contend with such a sudden and unexpected standstill – not even a gradual deceleration, but rather an abrupt and jarring emergency stop. Our velocentric lifestyles coupled with the increasing valorisation of resilience have led to our forgetting how to slow down. Often struggling to stay afloat amidst relentless waves of restless activity, we struggle to discover let alone rest in any oceanic feeling. Rather than reawakening any dormant desire for a more human and humane pace of life, the post-Covid age is gearing up to be a new age of even greater acceleration, an age where our machines, newly aided by generative artificial intelligence, may soon easily outpace and replace us. This raises a more pressing existential question, what to do with ourselves when we are inevitably outrun and left behind?

In the familiar terminology of Erich Fromm (2013), we have forgotten how to simply *be* and appear lost in ultimately meaningless and unsatisfying modes of *having*, with all their associated activities of acquiring. In the digital domain, we may frequently find ourselves compulsively consuming whilst actively parading our consumption for online audiences for reciprocal likes and validation.

In Fromm's (2001) posthumously published 'The Art of Being', he critiques the prevailing consumer culture of his day and prescribes the cultivation of stillness as an antidote to the prevailing restlessness, meaninglessness and monotony of modern life. The book provides examples of Fromm's emphasis on transcendence, deeply influenced by Zen Buddhism, its central message being:

> Read the writings of Masters of Living, learn to understand the true meaning of their words, form your own conviction of what you want to do with your life; and get over the naïve idea that you need no master, no guide, no model, that you can find out in a lifetime what the greatest minds of the human species have discovered in many thousands of years.
>
> *(Ibid., p. 9)*

Following in his spirit, *this* book seeks out and studies the *Masters of Slow Living*. For far too many have become far too accustomed to and accepting of the pathological pace of modern life, without recognising its increasingly costly toll on our health and well-being. In the following chapters, I intend to demonstrate what nourishing and transformative wisdom we can rediscover through slowing down and cultivating stillness.

To do this, I will need to return to the sources, the spiritual custodians of slow living – as found in some of the world's ancient living wisdom traditions. The cosmologies and psychologies of Hinduism, Buddhism, Daoism and Judaism provide precious templates for minds calmed and time reclaimed – consciously countering the 'cult of speed' (Honoré 2004). Through attending to these traditions, we may eventually recover a more reenchanted, purposeful and happier life, whilst reframing our thinking towards ecology and technology.

What follows is a cross-cultural, psychological and spiritual deep dive into a much-needed alternative, decelerated way of life.

References

Ackerman, S. (2017) Exploring Freud's resistance to the oceanic feeling. *Journal of the American Psychoanalytic Association*, 65(1), pp. 9–31.

Benson, C. (2001) *The Cultural Psychology of Self: Place, Morality and Art in Human Worlds*. London: Routledge.

Blake, W. (1893) *The Poems of William Blake* (Ed. Yeats, W. B.). London: Lawrence and Bullen.

Calhoun, J. (1970) Population density and social pathology. *California Medicine*, 113(5), p. 54

Chapman, T. (1988) *Fast Car*. Los Angeles: Elektra.

Cittaslow Manifesto. (2023) [Online]. Available at: www.cittaslow.org/content/cittaslow-manifesto (Accessed 22 February 2023).

Connor, M. and Armitage, C. (2002) *The Social Psychology of Food*. Buckingham: Open University Press.

Ford, H. (1921) *The International Jew – Volume 3*. Detroit: The Dearborn Publishing Company.

Forster, E. M. (2012) *The Machine Stops and Other Stories*. London: Pan Macmillan.

Fromm, E. (2001) *The Art of Being*. New York: Continuum.

Fromm, E. (2013) *To Have or to Be?* London: Bloomsbury Academic.

Gabaccia, D. (2009) *We Are What We Eat: Ethnic Food and the Making of Americans*. Cambridge, MA: Harvard University Press.

Gordon, A. and Suzuki, D. (1991) *It's a Matter of Survival*. Cambridge, MA: Harvard University Press.

Halberstam, D. (2003) Citizen ford. In: Wood, J. and Wood, M. (Eds.) *Henry Ford: Critical Evaluations in Business and Management*. London: Routledge, pp. 56–80.

Honoré, C. (2004) *In Praise of Slow: How a Worldwide Movement Is Challenging the Cult of Speed*. London: Harper Collins.

Laplanche, J. and Pontalis, J. (2004) *The Language of Psychoanalysis*. London: Karnac Books.

Marinetti, F. (1909) The futurist manifesto [Online]. Available at: http://bactra.org/T4PM/futurist-manifesto.html (Accessed 21 March 2023).

Marinetti, F. (2014) *The Futurist Cookbook*. London: Penguin.

Marx, K. (1990) *Capital: A Critique of Political Economy – Volume 1*. London: Penguin Books.

Nelson, M. (2022) *Excessivism* [Website]. Available at: www.excessivism.com (Accessed 22 February 2022).

Parkins, W. and Craig, G. (2006) *Slow Living*. New York: Berg.

Purser, R. (2019) *McMindfulness: How Mindfulness Became the New Capitalist Spirituality*. London: Repeater Books.

Ritzer, G. (2015) *The McDonaldisation of Society*. Thousand Oaks, CA: Sage Publications.

Ruler, P. (2010) *Ludlow and the Shropshire Hills: Ironbridge and the Severn Gorge*. Oxford: Chris Andrews Publications Ltd.

Ryle, M. and Soper, K. (2013) Alternative hedonism: The world by bicycle. In: Osbaldiston. N. (Ed.) *Culture of the Slow: Social Deceleration in an Accelerated World*. New York: Palgrave Macmillan, pp. 94–109.
Schulkin, J. (Ed.) (2004) *Allostasis, Homeostasis and the Costs of Physiological Adaptation*. Cambridge: Cambridge University Press.
Slosar, J. R. (2009) *The Culture of Excess: How America Lost Self-Control and Why We Need to Redefine Success*. Westport, CT: Greenwood Publishing.
The Henry Ford [Online]. Available at: www.thehenryford.org/collections-and-research/digital-resources/popular-topics/sociological-department (Accessed 23 June 2022).
Tuan, Y.-F. (1990) *Topophilia: A Study of Environmental Perception, Attitudes and Values*. New York: Columbia University Press.
Virilio, P. (1977) *Speed and Politics: An Essay on Dromology*. New York: Semitotexte.
Virilio, P. (2003) *Art and Fear*. London: Continuum.
Virilio, P. (2007) *Speed and Politics* (Trans. Polizzotti, T.). Los Angeles, CA: Semiotext(e).
Werness, H. (2006) *The Contiuum Encyclopedia of Animal Symbolism in Art*. New York: Continuum.
WHO (2022) COVID 19 pandemic triggers 25% increase in prevalence of anxiety and depression worldwide [Online]. Available at: www.who.int/news/item/02-03-2022-covid-19-pandemic-triggers-25-increase-in-prevalence-of-anxiety-and-depression-worldwide (Accessed 24 August 2022).

2

KALI YUGA

Living in the Age of Speed

My earliest introduction to Hindu thought and cosmology was through the writings of Alan Watts, one of the foremost popularisers of Eastern spirituality in the West. In Watts' (2002) 'The Tao of Philosophy', he reflected on the nature of time and of mind, and on the disenchanted, increasingly fragmented era we live in. In the second chapter, he briefly and somewhat irreverently introduces the traditional, cyclical Hindu view of time, discussing the duration of a *Kalpa* – totalling over four billion years, a little less than the estimated age of the Earth according to geologists.

A *Kalpa* is typically divided into four time periods, beginning with the longest *Satya Yuga*, or Age of Truth. This beginning is often described as being a glorious golden age due to its stability and humanity's clear perception of and closeness to Divine truth during this exalted era. But with each passing age that stability, perception and closeness become gradually more unstable, obscured and distant. The following ages of *Treta* and *Dvapara* become progressively shorter and faster as their proximity from the truth becomes farther:

> And finally comes the shortest period when everything bad triumphs, and the whole universe blows up and we begin all over again. We are supposed to be living in that period now. It is what is called the *Kali Yuga*, the Age of Darkness, and it began on Friday, February 23rd, 3123 B.C., and it has 5000 years to run. However, as it goes on, time gets faster, so do not worry.
>
> *(Watts 2002, p. 23)*

DOI: 10.4324/9781003334972-2

The fact that Watts had somehow settled on the day and month of my birth as marking the beginning of the end of days was personally disconcerting. Additionally, the observation that 'time gets faster' appears to be a genuine cause for concern rather than any source of consolation, as Gita Mehta had cautioned:

> The Indian myth maintains we are living in the age of Kalyug, which presages the end of the world. Kalyug is characterised by speed. Speed, being the enemy of reflection, will spread fantasy with such velocity that humans, in their pursuit of escape, will ultimately destroy themselves.
>
> *(Mehta 1994)*

Yet Watts, guided by the world view and wisdom of the Hindu *Vedas*, recognises that the inevitable conclusion is that 'we begin all over again', so that nothing is ultimately lost or gained. It is similar to one song ending before another begins, and as a popular Sanskrit saying recalls *Nāda Brahma* – the world is sound.

There even appears to be an auditory equivalent of the *yuga* cycle that can be heard within the traditional structure of Hindustani music (Simms 1992–1993). All pieces begin with stillness and silence, before the familiar, accompanying drone of the stringed *tanpura* begins, recollecting the timeless period prior to creation. The following section called *Alaap* is typically a slow, improvised, leisurely-played melody without accompanying percussion – it finds and makes its own pace, leading into the *Vilambitlaya*. In the *Vilambitlaya* cycle, one may introduce the familiar, regulating, cyclic rhythm of the *tabla*, called *taal*, that continues into the mid-paced *Madhyalaya*. *Drutlaya* is the final and fastest section, often where a musician demonstrates their capacity to play at astonishing speeds, displaying great virtuosity through dizzying, disorientating displays of musical mastery which the percussionist must somehow match. The racing pace of the composition leads to something approximating a sonic disintegration or dissolution, *Mahapralaya* – 'the Great Destruction' as encountered in the age of the *Kali Yuga*, typically concluding in a single, unified final note and beat that returns us back to the silence heard at the very beginning.

> So too is the disintegrated universe reintegrated into the Absolute during the Mahapralaya, only to begin again after an interval of a 'Night of Brahma' – Divine Play.
>
> *(Simms 1992–1993, p. 79)*

Watts too would often use the more playful language of music to critique our culture's outcome-driven, goal-obsessed way of living:

> In music one doesn't make the end of the composition the point of the composition. If that were so, the best conductors would be those who played fastest, and there would be composers who wrote only finales . . .

> We thought of life by analogy, with a journey, with a pilgrimage, which had a serious purpose at the end. The thing was to get to that end, success or whatever it is . . . But we missed the point the whole way along – it was a musical thing, and you were supposed to sing or dance while the music was being played.
>
> *(Watts 1965)*

Hindu thought understands there to be an inherent, divine play or *Lila* – that underscores and brings about both creation and destruction. According to one popular Hindu creation narrative, this entire reality (including this book you're currently holding) may simply be the vivid dream of the God Vishnu. Mistaking one's dream for reality and one's imaginings for the truth is frequently explored through the Vedic teachings in relation to *Maya*.

In Sanskrit, *Maya* typically refers to the pseudo, magical, illusory quality of our perception of the world, and how all too often we see only what we wish or expect to see, rather than what is truly there. A closely related term and concept is *Adhyāsa*, referring to our habitual tendency to project or superimpose assumed attributes onto ourselves, onto others and onto the various phenomena or stimuli we encounter. A popular example of *Adhyāsa* is of being in a dark room and mistaking a twisted pile of rope for a coiled, venomous snake – the rope remains a rope, the snake is simply imagined, but our mistaken perception and resultant fear response are immediate and intense. One may even die of fright! But then again, death itself is also ultimately understood to be an illusion, brought about by our ignorance of our true nature, which is, according to the Hindu scriptures, deathless and Divine. It is therefore ignorance, *Avidya*, that is the source of all our psychological and social suffering – particularly ignorance regarding the true, original nature of our own minds.

Vedantic Depth Psychology

My formal study of Hinduism, preceding my eventual sojourn in India, began at a Manchester Vedanta study circle, where Swamis would visit fortnightly to teach Sanskrit and instruct us in the Upanishads.

The very first Swami I met seemed particularly interested to learn that I was a psychologist and suggested that we were actually travelling upon similar paths, but respectfully observed that my study of the mind had stopped somewhat short – that I and my fellow psychologists had become far too preoccupied with the mere surface cognitions and transitory emotions while the true depths of our being remained unexplored.

Whereas I was a student of Psychology, the Swami clarified that he was a student of *Atmavidya*, the 'science of the Self' – the true, deeper and Divine Self – the *Atman*, which always remains, ever present, just behind, beneath or beyond our ordinary, everyday waking awareness. I took some pride in disclosing to the Swami that as a *Transpersonal*

Psychologist, I too was exploring mystical, non-ordinary and non-dual states of consciousness through contemplative practice, briefly mentioning the work of William James, Carl Jung, Abraham Maslow and Stanislav Grof for good measure.

In order to explore these Transpersonal themes further, we studied the *Upanishads*, classic Hindu scriptures that explore the relationship between *Atman* – the Self – and *Brahman* – the Divine underlying, ultimate reality. Ultimately *Atman* and *Brahman* are understood not to be two separate entities but actually one and the same being, but our ignorance of this reality results in much suffering and confusion until we may eventually seek out this union through spiritual disciplines and practices – in fact 'union', specifically with the Divine, is a literal translation of the now familiar term and ubiquitous practice of *Yoga*.

Perhaps it is no surprise that in the age of the Kali Yuga even Yoga appears typically stripped of its spiritual core and content, and is commonly reduced to being just another evening exercise class or mildly exotically Eastern recreational activity. A great many yoga classes' primary focus is often restricted to the outer, surface elements, on the bodily postures, forms and stretches – the *Asanas*, as opposed to any inner goal of awakening to a deeper, Divine reality.

It is worth recalling that in Patanjali's seminal text, the *Yoga Sutras* (Vivekananda 2011), the *Asanas* constitute only one part of an eightfold practice or 'limbs' of Yoga which culminates in *Samadhi* – the transcending of one's ordinary sense of self, a purification of one's polluted and partial perception, leading to an awakened realisation of an uninterrupted unity with Divinity. Our fixation on the outer postures may distract us from the inner purpose; the excessive focus on one limb to the virtual exclusion of all the others makes for an incomplete and unstable practice, but then again fragmentariness and instability are both hallmarks of the present age. During the Kali Yuga, we seem to become increasingly mired in *Maya*, losing our capacity to discern truth from fiction and what is fundamental from what is peripheral.

This gradual loss of clarity and stability is vividly described in the Hindu scripture *Śrimad Bhāgavatam* (Prabhupāda 2017) where the Hindu Dharma is compared, in the golden age, to a sturdy bull, standing firm on the four legs of austerity, cleanliness, compassion and truthfulness. With each passing age, the bull loses a leg becoming increasingly unbalanced – in our final age, the bull is precariously balanced on just one solitary, increasingly strained and shaky leg of truth.

And so the last leg is truth, and truth appears to be on its last legs. It seems particularly pertinent that our age is increasingly referred to as being the age of 'post-truth' – fake news and deep fakes, a time of confusion, contradictions and competing conspiracies, fuelled by deepening mutual mistrusts and the proliferation of misinformation. One might even say that the bull of

Dharma has long since departed and we are now wading together through an age of 'bullshit' (Frankfurt 2005).

In addition to being legless, this modern age may also be 'headless', according to the esteemed Ceylonese philosopher and historian Ananda Coomaraswamy, who was one of the first writers to introduce Hindu and Buddhist thought to the West:

> Modern civilization, by its divorce from any principle, can be likened to a headless corpse of which the last motions are convulsive and insignificant.
> *(Coomaraswamy quoted in Fitzgerald and Singam 2011, p. 13)*

Although seemingly bleak and hopeless, if one were to take a more Tantric view and interpretation of this apparently grotesque image, a more optimistic and potentially significant and salvational message may be gleamed.

Tantra represents and advocates a more esoteric, often antinomian, seemingly transgressive path to union with the Divine (Ramos 2020). With the guidance of a qualified Guru, one learns to transform and transmute the powerful, potentially destructive, sexual and aggressive drives into the very fuel for reaching awakening. The more famous and infamous acts of various Tantric gurus in both Hindu and Buddhist contexts may be purposefully shocking in order to jolt a practitioner out of their *samsaric* stupor. What to the uninitiated might appear as the abandoning of more normative principles and practices may actually be an expression of non-dual awareness – a seeing and being beyond more orthodox, dualistic categories and dichotomies of pure versus impure, good versus evil, awakened versus deluded. This can also be viscerally encountered in the often startling iconography of Tantra.

The Hindu Goddess *Chhinnamasta*, a tantric incarnation of the Divine Feminine principle, is traditionally, graphically depicted in the very act of decapitating herself whilst ecstatically dancing. In this instance, the severed head symbolises the death of ego, the transcending of self-centredness, unleashing and leading to great power and Self-realisation. The imagery may appear somewhat shocking and extreme, but one might justifiably argue that we are living in shocking and extreme times, one in which tantric methods may be particularly appropriate and effective. So, even in the midst of the Kali Yuga, there still appears to be the possibility of salvation.

Drawing Closer

As our distance from the golden age increases, we grow increasingly distant from truth, even losing our ability to discern the truth; we lose its thread and consequently lose our way. It is significant therefore that the title of the scriptures, *Upanishads*, literally means to draw nearer to – nearer to both one's Guru and to the truth.

The *Upanishads* underpin and inform the *Advaita Vedanta* tradition – *Advaita* referring to non-duality and *Vedanta* referring to the culmination of knowledge concerning the Divine. *Advaita Vedanta* was popularised in the West by the esteemed Swami Vivekananda, who notably addressed the World Parliament of Religions in 1893, to much acclaim and enduring admiration.

Vivekananda was keen to communicate the depth, breadth and sophistication of Hindu thought and practice, and to counter any lingering colonialist myths and misinformation concerning Indian religion being primitive or superstitious. Yoga in particular, he repeatedly explained, is an advanced form of inner science, the original and superior Psychology (Vivekananda 2007). In so explaining, he sought to demonstrate India's ability and inborn right to self-govern.

His erudite presentation of *Vedanta* demonstrated that whilst the West was unquestionably far ahead in regard to technological advancement and innovation, when compared to the East, it appeared spiritually impoverished.

To his fellow Indian advocates of home rule and critics of British colonialism, the Western Psyche wasn't merely excessively materialist, it was potentially destructive. In particular, the Western preoccupation with speed and productivity was noted as having a psychologically detrimental, dehumanising and despiritualising effect on humankind.

Mahatma Gandhi's critiques of colonialism were as much concerned with reclaiming and reaffirming the need for spiritual self-realisation as they were with achieving political self-determination. Gandhi's primary preoccupation was with the truth, and his search for and sincere efforts to embody this truth. This quest is explored throughout his autobiography, first published in 1925, which bore the alternate title 'The Story of My Experiments with Truth' (Gandhi 2003).

When it came to his fight against the British Empire, it was truth itself that Gandhi sought to weaponise – his particular form of non-violent protest was originally termed *Satyagraha* – literally holding firmly to truth, and its advocates known collectively as *Satyagrahis*.

The violent and very public assault of hundreds of unarmed *Satyagrahis* at the Dharsana Salt Works in 1930, who were peacefully but persistently protesting against the unjust British salt tax, was one such event that was intended to expose the true face of imperialism.

The abiding iconography of Gandhi depicts him sitting, dressed simply in a *dhoti*, before a simply wooden *charkha* (spinning wheel), fully immersed in the activity of spinning cotton thread – leading by example, personifying and figure-heading his national homespun movement.

The striking contrast between early photographs of Mr Mohandas K Gandhi attorney at law, a serious and seemingly loyal subject of the British empire, dressed in the manner of an English gentleman and the later photographs of a smiling old man, a sparsely-attired *Mahatma* (great soul), visually attested to his spiritual and psychological rebirth. A younger Winston Churchill cynically scoffed at this transformation by referring to Gandhi as a 'seditious fakir, striding half-naked up the steps of the Viceroy's palace to negotiate with the representative of the King-Emperor' (Churchill quoted in Erikson 1993, p. 447). However, he had quite unintentionally flattered Gandhi, who ardently aspired to be a *Fakir* – a true renunciate and seeker of truth. Gandhi's philosophy and movement represented a robust renunciation of modernity with its technocentric lifestyles and multiplying desires, in essence, he advocated a return to slow living:

> If I preach against the modern artificial life of sensual enjoyment, and ask men and women to go back to the simple life epitomised in the *charkha*, I do so because I know without an intelligent return to simplicity, there is no escape from our descent to a state lower than brutality.
>
> *(Gandhi quoted in Chakrabarti 2000, p. 13)*

The wheel itself is and remains a perennial symbol of human progress from the advent of the first wheel around 4000 BCE, to chariots, then carriages, leading up to today's automobiles, or to the mechanised wheels and turbines of modern industry. Gandhi's wooden wheel, by contrast, emphasises autonomy and conscious intention over efficiency and automation.

At the centre of the flag of India, one still finds the *Ashoka Chakra*, named after the great Buddhist emperor of India, symbolising the eternal wheel of truth. Rather than signifying technological progress, the *Chakra* traditionally conveys spiritual potential and evolution.

In many Yogic systems, and also amongst many New Age adherents, this is illustrated in the well-known representation of the seven inner *Chakras* – psycho-spiritual centres located within and culminating just above the human frame. These seven centres relate to one's level of spiritual and psychological awareness and attainment, beginning at the physical, material base of the spine, ascending above the crown of the head into the *Sahasrāra* – thousand-petalled lotus, denoting spiritual awakening.

The lotus is commonly used in both Hindu and Buddhist iconography to represent the inner alchemy of spiritual practice. The lotus often grows in the muddy, stagnant pond yet emerges above the surface, opening untouched and unblemished. As a psychospiritual symbol, the lotus reminds and reassures us that even in the midst of all the mud of *maya* (or the 'bullshit') we may still awaken and recollect our Divine connection and consciousness. Like the physical lotus flower, the *Sahasrāra Charka* is raised just above the head, directing us towards something beyond the material world of matter.

The symbolism of and sentiment behind the wheel persists today at Gandhi's ashram at Sabarmati in Ahmedabad, India. When former US President Donald Trump was taken on a tour of the ashram by Indian Prime Minister

Modi in 2000, both President Trump and the First Lady were filmed visiting the iconic charkha. The sight of the 'leader of the free world', a man widely known for, even celebrated for his brashness and impulsivity, hailing from a land whose popular mantra is 'Bigger, Better, Faster, Newer', standing by the simple wooden wheel made for a striking and incongruous scene.

The practical act of spinning cotton itself requires a great degree of skill and patience – one's attention needs to be gently yet fully focused on the task at hand. One's motions must be smooth and subtle; one should resist the familiar temptation to forcefully pull at the cotton, but instead firmly hold as one spins to avoid knotting or tearing. Ideally, when spinning cotton on the charkha, there should be harmony between one's movements, attention to one's breath and intentions, in order to synchronise oneself with the slow and steady rhythm of the practice. Indeed, spinning cotton at a charkha could be considered mindfulness in motion.

The Indian homespun movement was not simply about countering the detrimental economic, political and social impact of importing mass-produced cotton from the mechanised mills of Leeds and Manchester but represented a renunciation of mass industrialisation and the mounting mechanisation of mankind, a pacifistic protest against the violent, colonialist and contagious cultures of speed and greed. For Gandhi, the West had come to embody some of the very darkest attributes of the Kali Yuga, and he sincerely believed that the hope for any future salvation may one day depend on the East (specifically India) preserving its rural traditions and remembering its spiritual heritage.

One of Gandhi's contemporaries, the Indian nationalist, philosopher, Guru and pioneer of Integral Yoga, Sri Aurobindo, would present a more sympathetic and cautiously optimistic vision of humankind's potential future spiritual evolution.

Alongside humankind's physical and technological evolutions, Aurobindo outlined a process which he termed involution. Involution described the gradual descent of spirit into matter, until spirit and spirituality are seemingly eclipsed by or consumed within materialism.

This involutionary process has a clear parallel in another description of the progression of the *yugas* being classified in relation to particular metals described in the encyclopaedic *Puranas* – with the first *Satya* age of truth being gold, followed by the silver *Treta Yuga* and the bronze *Dwapara Yuga*. Each metal represents an increasing heaviness, a deepening descent into density and darkness – ending in our *Kali Yuga*, the age of iron. Indeed, the relationship between iron and industry, from the first emergence of crude iron tools to the industrial revolution may appear self-evident.

Aurobindo perceived an underlying, organising and guiding Divine principle, arguing that our modern age suffered primarily from an immature, incorrect channelling or misapplication of our collective creative forces which were unconsciously impeding our spiritual evolution.

The West in particular had focused excessively on the surface of things, hampered by a myopic materialist mindset, in pursuit of a mere 'surface vitalism' (Aurobindo quoted in McDermott 2001, p. 196) alongside a denial of spirit that prevented any deeper sense of meaning or discovery of our original transcendent nature and purpose.

While commenting on the industrialisation of the nineteenth century and the destructive wars of the twentieth century, Aurobindo reflects:

> The vital élan brought us no deliverance, but only used the machinery already created with more feverish insistence, a vehement attempt to live more rapidly, more intensely, an inordinate will to act and to succeed, to enlarge the mere force of living, to pile up a gigantic efficiency of life.
>
> *(Ibid., p. 196)*

For Aurobindo, we risk becoming mere cogs in the wheels of a vast soulless machine whose only real purpose is to produce evermore cogs.

Aurobindo's solution was Integral Yoga, a way to meaningfully recover, reawaken and reinvigorate our spiritual core, and then to infuse and reintegrate our material form with spiritual substance and being. For Aurobindo (as with Vivekananda before him), Yoga was understood to be a deeper form of practical psychology (Banerji 2020), one which should incorporate Vedic, Tantric and scientific methods, with the conscious intention to extend beyond our ordinary surface, consensus consciousness into the recovery of what he termed the Supermind.

Through Integral Yoga one is seeking to consciously reconnect with the still, silent, original core of our inner being and rediscover our Divine nature. Whereas mainstream Psychology tends to focus on the cognitive contents of consciousness, Aurobindo emphasised the necessity to familiarise ourselves with our *transcognitive* capacities:

> There is nothing mind can do that cannot be done better by the mind's immobility and thought-free stillness.
>
> When mind is still, then Truth gets her chance to be heard in the purity of the silence.
>
> Truth cannot be attained by the Mind's thought but only by identity and silent vision. Truth lives in the calm wordless light of the eternal spaces; she does not intervene in the cackle of logical debate.
>
> *(Aurobindo quoted in McDermott 2001, p. 68)*

Such a view has its source in the Upanishads.

Finding Truth through Stillness

Our Manchester Vedanta study circle began with an in-depth study of the third chapter, first verse of the *Mundaka Upanishad*, which begins:

> Two birds, companions and friends,
> Cling to the same tree.
> One of them eats the sweet pippala-berry,
> The other looks on without eating.
> (Roebuck 2003, p. 327)

The Swami assured us that this seemingly simple and short verse contained a very profound teaching. At present, we are much like the first bird, busily occupying itself at the lower part of the tree – singing for a mate, busily building and reinforcing our nests, and seeking out the sweet fruit. This first bird appears lost in activity, thoughts and feelings – ensnared and ultimately exhausted by the world of endless distractions and competing sense pleasures. By contrast, the second bird sits aloft in the upper branches, silently observing and witnessing, utterly content in their stillness.

This first bird is arguably the one we are most intimately familiar with and that is studied by contemporary, mainstream psychologists – the everyday consensus consciousness, our vast array of thoughts, feelings and behaviours that correspond and contribute to our sense of self. This is the familiar self that seeks security, happiness and meaning, love and belonging; the self that has dreams, fears and aspirations. This is also the self that seeks pleasure, the hedonic pleasures of senses – frequently, 'naturally' seeking excitement, novelty and entertainment. To seek such pleasure is indeed the norm, for not to do so risks placing one in a more psychopathological frame – consider the clinical term anhedonia, referring to the individual who doesn't actively seek out or experience pleasure and may consequently be diagnosed as depressed or otherwise psychologically dysfunctional. This diagnostic term may be problematic if inappropriately applied to a spiritual practitioner who seeks something beyond the hedonic treadmill, and consciously renounces the so-called worldly pleasures.

The very term *Mundaka* from the *Mundaka Upanishad* traditionally refers to a shaven-headed ascetic, an ancient and still-living tradition of renunciation, referring to spiritual practitioners who saw through and consequently, intentionally eschew a life of hedonic fulfilment, in order to seek something deeper, something that transcends our ordinary concepts of pain and pleasure, loss and gain, delight and regret.

The Swami explained that the first bird will eventually inevitably tire, as desires are endless and ultimately impossible to satisfy in any lasting, meaningful sense. Partly through exhaustion, perhaps desperation, the first bird longingly gazes at the second bird still peacefully perched in the upper branches, and gradually begins to ascend. Upon eventually reaching the upper branches, the reunion of the two birds leads to a blissful union as the previous duality of perceiver and perceived dissolves – there is only and was only ever one bird.

The Italian Psychiatrist and founder of Psychosynthesis, Roberto Assagioli, had also been guided by the *Upanishads*, and presented a meditative exercise intended to elicit this transpersonal state through what he termed 'dis-identification' (Assagioli 2000, p. 103). The purpose of dis-identification is to observe the transient and partial nature of what we commonly refer to as self – noting how we typically over-identify with our physicality, thoughts and feelings. Assagioli encourages us to observe that although we *have* a body, we are not reducible *to* this body – thus he begins by challenging our fixation on the physical, our over-identification with the body:

> The first step is to affirm with conviction and to become aware of the fact that: 'I *have* a body, but I *am not* my body.' That seems evident. This body is something material and changeable (it has been stated that within a few years all the cells of the body are renewed). Nevertheless, we mistakenly identify ourselves all the time with our body and attribute to the 'I' all our physical sensations.
>
> *(Ibid.)*

One proceeds likewise with one's thoughts and emotions, each time recognising their inherent changeability and instability. This inevitably leads one into a state of aporia and to the question – if I am not my body, thoughts or feelings, then *what* or *who* am *I*?

If we consider and meditate upon the message of *Mundaka Upanishad*, we may well consider to what extent we too are lost in the busyness of the first bird – habitually, compulsively consuming the sweet pippala berries. It appears that the world is set up in such a way to keep us moving ever faster towards some unstated, ambiguous goal that keeps moving just out of reach.

Acceleration and consumption appear to be two defining features of our age. Consuming to the point where we ourselves are consumed. Speeding towards our final destination only to discover that the final destination was speed itself.

The Psychology of the Kali Yuga

Marty Glass's (2001) 'Yuga: An Anatomy of Our Fate' is an engaging, at times disorientating stream of consciousness, exploring and critiquing our increasingly precarious age. As a former student of the great comparative theologian Huston Smith, Glass is keen to note how this apocalyptic mindset with its eschatological expectations is not the sole reserve of Hinduism but is shared amongst a great many world faiths. Even those of a more secular disposition may justifiably share a sense of impending doom. In a sobering example of synchronicity, as I began writing this chapter, on January 24, 2022, The Bulletin of the Atomic Scientists moved the Doomsday clock ninety seconds to midnight, the closest it has ever been since its inception in 1947. Initially, the clock was set at seven minutes to midnight in view of the risk of nuclear conflict and mutually assured destruction, but has since widened the scope of world-ending catastrophes to include climate change and global pandemics.

For some centuries, Christian theologians have been looking for, and increasingly easily finding evidence that we are living through the 'End Times', just prior to the final 'Day of Judgement'. Evangelical pastors abound, proclaiming the advent of the age of the anti-Christ – decrying the decadent and immoral times we inhabit. Islamic eschatology, discussed in the *Hadiths*, likewise anticipates the widespread abandonment of morality and decency, coupled with a rise in ecological disasters that sound concerningly close to the evermore frequent reports of extreme weather events occurring around the globe. Buddhists also consider this age to be the 'Dharma Ending Age' where confusion will abound as to the true teachings of the Buddha, when subsequently the paths to and opportunities for awakening and liberation will become increasingly unclear and rare.

Glass identifies five main characteristics that typify the *Kali Yuga* which one might observe, sound eerily similar to the process of McDonaldisation – the fall into time, the reign of quantity, the mutation into machinery, the end of nature and the prison of unreality:

> Time speeds up in the *Kali-Yuga*, the cosmic substance flows ever faster. Electric cities, electric lives, it's a speed-of-light nanosecond cyber-world now; the minutes close like clamps upon our blurred hurrying, step on it, it's getting late; wires and grids, unintelligible techno-terms acronymized so you can say them faster, the Great International Telecommunications Web, the super-charged ground and air humming and writhing with pulses of money, money and information, money and information racing the digital clocks through the metallic voids, through the intercontinental cyber-space: the goal is always instantaneous.
>
> *(Glass 2001, p. 119)*

A central theme throughout Glass's thesis is the prevailing disenchantment with and desacralisation of our world, leading to a firm yet flawed fixation with the material and measurable. This appears to have its counterpart, a parallel process, occurring within the history of Psychology and Psychotherapy, to the extent that we might ask to what extent is contemporary Psychology itself a by-product of the Kali Yuga?

The birth of both Psychology and Psychotherapy is often attributed to Freud's Psychoanalytic tradition, also known as depth psychology – often termed the First Force by historians of psychology. This was a revolutionary approach for the time, introducing many to the role of the unconscious in daily life. However, Freud's originality and genius were often overshadowed by his pessimistic view of people; at times he appears to despair of the violence and destructive capacities inherent in human nature:

> Men are not gentle creatures, who want to be loved, who at the most can defend themselves if they are attacked; they are, on the contrary, creatures among whose instinctual endowments is to be reckoned a powerful share of aggressiveness. As a result, their neighbour is for them not only a potential helper or sexual object, but also someone who tempts them to satisfy their aggressiveness on him, to exploit his capacity for work without compensation, to use him sexually without his consent, to seize his possessions, to humiliate him, to cause him pain, to torture and to kill him. *Homo homini lupus* [man is wolf to man]. Who in the face of all his experience of life and of history, will have the courage to dispute this assertion?
>
> *(Freud 1961, pp. 58–59)*

Consequently, depth psychology frequently appears to focus on the brutish depths that human beings may sink to, as opposed to any humane heights that they might aspire or ascend to. For Freud, human beings' basic nature is barbaric; we seek protection and reassurance behind the thin façades of civilisation and culture – all the while remaining dangerously unaware of and pulled along by the powerful, unseen currents of the unconscious.

Our Psyche is envisioned as a battleground, where we are beleaguered by sexual and aggressive drives. There is no sense or promise of redemption, no spiritual salvation or salve in some 'oceanic feeling' or guiding light; one may only become more aware of rising darkness and seek to steel oneself against it. Freud perceives and offers no spiritual awakening, no final *Ananda* or bliss, only the achievement or acceptance of 'common unhappiness' as opposed to 'hysterical misery' (Freud and Breuer 1999, p. 351). There is also arguably an apocalyptic reading of Freud's work, particularly in relation to his discussion of the death drive and Nirvana principle – that hidden behind all our protestations concerning the sanctity of life and the pressing need to nurture and preserve it, we may secretly yearn for oblivion.

One colleague who quite defiantly opposed Freud's bleak assessment of humanity was Carl Jung, whom Freud had once sincerely hoped would inherit the mantle of the Psychoanalytic Society. Sensing Jung's interest in all matters mystical, he had previously warned him away from the 'black mud of the occult' (Jung 1961, p. 150), without realising the extent to which Jung was already deeply immersed in metaphysical speculation and introspection in his sincere, lifelong quest for the numinous.

In stark contrast to Freud's Psychoanalysis, Jung's Analytical Psychology was profoundly spiritually charged – the world with all its mysteries, symbols and seeming coincidences was suffused, indeed saturated with meaning and purpose. In Jung's 'Red Book' (Jung and Shamdasani 2009), one glimpses something of the extent of his esoteric pursuits through his encounters with the archetypes. Beyond Freud's personal unconscious, Jung had discovered and was keenly exploring and charting a collective unconscious – a reservoir of primordial forms and repository of ancient wisdom, populated by gods and goddesses, angels and demons, the heroes and monsters of all ages and cultures. Jung understood that much, if not all our personal and collective neuroses, was largely due to our ongoing repression and stubborn denial of this living spiritual reality, which for millennia had sustained us, offering deeper meaning and connection to ourselves, each other, and our world.

In 1958, three years before his death, Carl Jung published his classic 'The Undiscovered Self' which contained this sombre warning:

> A mood of universal destruction and renewal has set its mark on our age. This mood makes itself felt everywhere, politically, socially, and philosophically. We are living in what the Greeks called the *kairos* – the right moment for a 'metamorphosis of the gods,' of the fundamental principles and symbols. This peculiarity of our time, which is certainly not of our conscious choosing, is the expression of the unconscious human within us who is changing. Coming generations will have to take account of this momentous transformation if humanity is not to destroy itself through the might of its own technology and science.
>
> *(Jung quoted in Tarnas 1991, p. 412)*

When confronted with the threatening otherness of the unconscious, or the apparent chaos of the collective unconscious, it is perhaps little wonder that many psychologists sought solace in the comparative safety and order of the laboratory.

The Second Force of Behaviourism could trace their lineage back to the earlier experimental psychology of Wilhelm Wundt, who had established the first psychological laboratories in Leipzig in 1879 (three years before Freud began his medical career). The Behaviourists enthusiastically endorsed and emulated the empirical, experimental methods of the natural sciences. The messiness of introspection and subjectivity was replaced by direct empirical observation of behaviour with aspirations of objective measurement with the promise of predictive power. In its more radical forms, Behaviourism pursued a reductionist and deterministic path, as the richness and diversity of human experience were essentially reduced to an equation and acronym S→R, Stimulus and Response. In their pursuit of order and clarity, Behaviourism in general and B. F. Skinner, in particular, imagined themselves to be the final nail in the coffin of any lingering metaphysical or vitalist speculations that risked undermining the psychological sciences, instead adopting more mechanistic explanations:

> Man is a machine, but he is a very complex one. At present he is far beyond the powers of men to construct – except, of course, in the usual biological way. Only those who believe that something nonphysical is essential to his functioning are likely to question this.
>
> *(Skinner 1969, p. 294)*

In Behaviourism, we might detect the beginnings of a 'mutation into machinery' that the later Cognitive revolution would soon continue apace with far greater success.

Caught between a double determinism, the Scylla of the unconscious and the Charybdis of conditioning, Abraham Maslow earnestly sought a third way. The Third Force of Humanistic Psychology sought to recover a more human and humane approach to the burgeoning Psychological sciences. In part fuelled and informed by the optimism of 1960s counterculture and the Human Potential Movement, Maslow consciously moved away from models that psychopathologised and mechanised, shifting his attention to deeper questions of human meaning and purpose – peak experiences, self-actualisation, leading eventually to self-transcendence and the identification of a Fourth Force – Transpersonal Psychology.

In many ways, Maslow's work may be thought of as a return to the roots of American Psychology, particularly one of its most celebrated pioneers William James. It was James who gifted us with the term 'stream of thought' (James 1890, p. 224), frequently rephrased as a 'stream of consciousness' in his seminal text 'Principles of Psychology', and who also encouraged his students and peers to seriously investigate both the value and 'Varieties of Religious Experience' (1902).

Maslow's approach was to become profoundly influenced by spiritual teachings, particularly the Chinese tradition of Daoism. Maslow viewed Psychology and the deterministic models that underpinned it as having become too controlling and dehumanising to be helpful, instead promoting more Humanistic and Transpersonal approaches (Maslow 1993).

Today, one might notice that both Humanistic and Transpersonal Psychology have been largely relegated to the periphery of the discipline. Mainstream definitions of Psychology most commonly describe it as a 'Science of Mind and Behaviour' (Gross 2020).

Perhaps no other discipline has so closely followed the advice of Galileo Galilei to 'Measure what can be measured and make measurable what cannot be measured' (quoted in Dunn 2010, p. 57). The popular and highly profitable field of psychometrics (Furr and Bacharach 2008), replete with its ever-expanding batteries of tests, seeks to concretise and quantify the various elements of our personality – conveniently divided into measurable types or traits – with the Big Five remaining openness, conscientiousness, extraversion, agreeableness and neuroticism (known by the acronym OCEAN). With the advent of big data and assistance of machine-learning algorithms, newer competing models are emerging that claim even greater accuracy and predictive power (Tay et al. 2020). Psychometrics with its central roles in job candidate recruitment and clinical assessment, today constitutes an entire global industry, a convincing demonstration of the 'reign of quantity' (Glass 2001).

The involution of Psychology continues apace, as materialist approaches and positivist paradigms, particularly the cognitive and neuropsychological, appear to retain a firm hegemonic hold on the discipline. These approaches also appear to be far more easily adapted and transferred to digital domains. New Psychological disciplines such as Cyberpsychology are emerging in response to the rapidly rising tide of generative artificial intelligence, as our built and natural environments become ever more augmented and virtual. It might at first appear that the final two phases of the Kali Yuga, 'the end of nature and the prison of unreality' (Glass 2001), are upon us, but there are also signs that more Humanistic and Transpersonal yearnings are cautiously reasserting themselves – perhaps a return of the repressed.

Third wave approaches in Cognitive Therapy have also come to prominence over the last decade. Whilst they may at first appear to fit comfortably alongside the more mechanistic models of behavioural modification, with their impersonal and technical sounding acronyms DBT (Dialectical Behaviour Therapy), MBST (mindfulness-based stress reduction), MBCT (Mindfulness-Based Cognitive Therapy), and ACT (Acceptance Commitment Therapy), each one has its roots firmly planted in Eastern contemplative traditions, most typically Buddhism. Psychology and Psychotherapy appear to have made a space for stillness, although for now it remains a cautiously secular space.

It appears that the forces or ages of Psychology, much like the movements of time in Hindu cosmology, are also not linear but cyclical – first running from before returning to the spiritual. From a Hindu perspective, until we move towards a broader view of self which incorporates spirit – an *Atmavidya* – psychology will remain simply the study of our psychological surfaces. We will be content to continue observing the rise and fall of cognitive waves upon a largely unseen and unacknowledged Transpersonal ocean.

References

Assagioli, R. (2000) *Psychosynthesis: A Collection of Basic Writings*. Amherst, MA: The Synthesis Centre Inc.

Banerji, D. (Ed.) (2020) *Integral Yoga Psychology: Metaphysics and Transformation as Taught by Sri Aurobindo*. Twin Lakes, WI: Lotus Press.

Chakrabarti, M. (2000) *The Gandhian Philosophy of the Spinning Wheel*. New Delhi: Concept Publishing.

Dunn, P. (2010) *Measurement and Data Analysis for Engineering and Science*. Boca Raton, FL: CRC Press.
Erikson, E. H. (1993) *Gandhi's Truth: On the Origins of Militant Nonviolence*. New York: W.W. Norton.
Fitzgerald, J. and Singam, N. (Eds.) (2011) *The Wisdom of Ananda Coomaraswamy: Reflections on Indian Art, Life, and Religion*. Bloomington, IN: World Wisdom.
Frankfurt, H. G. (2005) *On Bullshit*. Princeton, NJ: Princeton University Press.
Freud, S. (1961) *Civilisation and Its Discontents*. New York: W.W. Norton.
Freud, S. and Breuer, J. (1999) *Studies on Hysteria*. London: Penguin Books.
Furr, R. M. and Bacharach, V. R. (2008) *Psychometrics: An Introduction*. London: Sage.
Gandhi, M. K. (2003) *An Autobiography, or, the Story of My Experiments with Truth*. Ahmedabad: Navajivan Publishing House.
Glass, M. (2001) *Yuga: An Anatomy of Our Fate*. Hillsdale, NY: Sophia Perennis.
Gross, R. (2020) *Psychology: The Science of Mind and Behaviour*. London: Hodder Education.
James, W. (1890) *The Principles of Psychology – Volume I*. New York: Henry Holt and Company.
James, W. (1902) *The Varieties of Religious Experience: A Study in Human Nature*. New York: Modern Library.
Jung, C. G. (1961) *Memories, Dreams, Reflections*. New York: Pantheon.
Jung, C. G. and Shamdasani, S. (Eds.) (2009) *The Red Book: Liber Novus*. New York: W.W. Norton.
Maslow, A. (1993) *Farther Reaches of Human Nature*. New York: Penguin Arkana.
McDermott, R. (2001) *The Essential Aurobindo: Writings of Sri Aurobindo*. MA: Lindisfarne Books.
Mehta, G. (1994) *Karma Cola*. Herndon, VA, London: Minerva.
Prabhupāda, A. C. B. (Trans.) (2017) *Śrimad Bhāgavatam – Ten Volume Set*. Mumbai: Krishna Books Incorporated.
Ramos, I. (2020) *Tantra: Enlightenment to Revolution*. New York: W. W. Norton.
Roebuck, V. (2003) *The Upanishads*. London: Penguin Books.
Simms, R. (1992–1993) Aspects of cosmological symbolism in Hindusthani musical forms. *Asian Music*, 24(1), pp. 67–89.
Skinner, B. F. (1969) *Contingencies of Reinforcement: A Theoretical Analysis*. New York: Applenton-Century-Crofts.
Tarnas, R. (1991) *The Passion of the Western Mind: Understanding the Ideas That Have Shaped Our World View*. New York: Harmony Books.
Tay, L., Proctor, R. and Woo, S. (2020) *Big Data in Psychological Research*. Washington, DC: American Psychological Association.
Vivekananda, S. (2007) *The Complete Works of Swami Vivekananda – Volume 2*. Kolkata: Advaita Ashrana.
Vivekananda, S. (Trans.) (2011) *The Yoga Sutras of Patanjali: The Essential Yoga Texts for Spiritual Enlightenment*. London: Watkins.
Watts, A. (1965) Lecture 1.1.4 – coincidence of opposites. Be here now network [Online]. Available at: https://beherenownetwork.com/alan-watts-being-in-the-way-ep-16-a-coincidence-of-opposites/ (Accessed 22 February 2023).
Watts, A. (2002) *The Tao of Philosophy*. Boston, MA: Tuttle Publishing.

3

CITTA SLOW

Settling the Mindstream

In previous chapters, we have kept revisiting the image of the wheel – from the spinning wheels of mechanised industry, the speeding wheels of automobiles, to the slower wooden wheels of cotton spinning *charkas*, and even to the more yogic, mystical inner wheels of ascending *chakras*. The wheel is also a prominent and reoccurring motif in Buddhist teachings and iconography.

When one enters a Buddhist temple, one will likely encounter the iconic and colourful *Bhavacakra*, 'Wheel of Life', or more literally the wheel of becoming. Typically, a mural, painting or Tibetan *thangka* of large wheel consisting of six realms, diversely populated by various beings, firmly held by Yama, the fanged Lord of death. This mandala-like depiction of *Samsaric* existence serves as a mnemonic map, allowing one to more easily navigate Buddhist cosmology and psychology.

Saṃsāra traditionally refers to the endless cycles of birth and death, as the term's etymology conveys the sense of revolving and turning. *Saṃsāra* is the monstrous monotony of being condemned to return and repeat life after life, each one marked and marred by suffering, impermanence, and a mistaken sense of self.

According to the Buddhist teachings, so much of our suffering is brought about due to our insistence that the world be other than it truly is. We habitually seek comfort in an imaginary sense of permanence, often resisting and recoiling from change. Yet our experience teaches us that everything inevitably changes – our world, our relationships even our sense and understanding of who we are. The Buddhist teachings refer to this reality as *Anicca* impermanence (Nyanatiloka 1997), more literally non-constant.

Our world, which at first glance seems so solid and abiding, is in a constant state of flux. Through the comparative lens of geological time, mountains rise

DOI: 10.4324/9781003334972-3

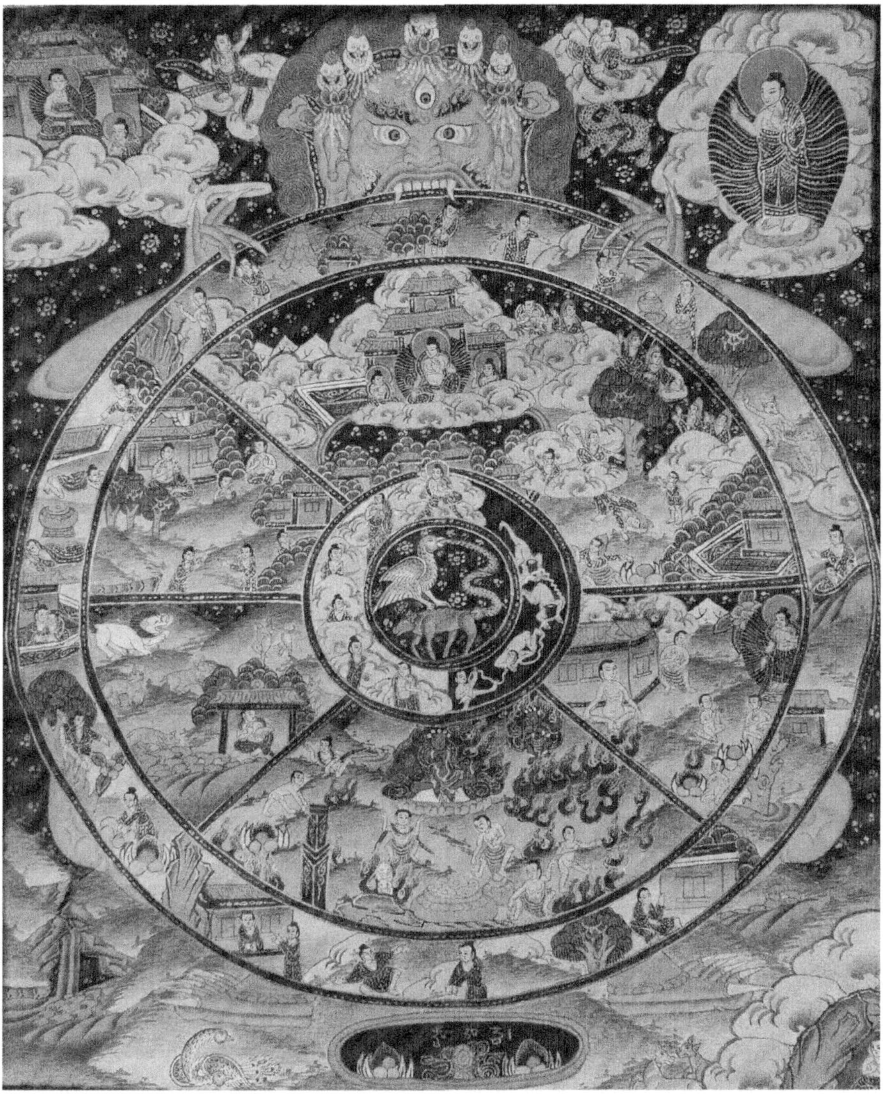

FIGURE 3.1 *Hand-painted Wheel of Life – Tibetan thangka from the author's private collection*

and fall like waves in a vast ocean. Even the stars, our familiar and comforting constellations, will one day exhaust their core supply of hydrogen and be extinguished. We likewise must all encounter the existential challenge of our own mortality, our own personal impermanence – but Buddhism goes further to interrogate *who* or *what* is actually born, lives and dies in the first instance.

We typically perceive and subsequently assume a relatively solid and stable sense of identity and continuity. Meditative practice reveals this to be simply an assumption. With more mindful introspection, we may come to realise that what we call self is in fact an ever-changing matrix of physical sensations, memories, emotions, relationships, hopes and fears, likes and dislikes – referred to in Buddhist terminology as *khandha*; commonly translated as aggregates, the various bundles that make up our being (Nyanatiloka 1997).

When we examine these aggregates more closely, we come to see that what we previously thought of as a coherent, autonomous being, experiencing our existence is actually *Anattā* – not-self. This term refers to a pseudo-sense of self, like a projection or mirage. This misperception works in much the same way as the familiar Gestalt effects, where a series of separate dots can appear to create a coherent circle, or the negative space within a geometric pattern convincingly suggests the presence of a triangle. But I would also propose that it is the *movement* and *motions* of this matrix, the various, dynamic patterns of thoughts and feelings that constitute our stream of consciousness, which imbue it with such a convincing reality. This is not too dissimilar from the way we are able to suspend disbelief and emotionally invest in an animated cartoon character, whose reality is simulated via the optical illusion of visually similar frames moving in quick succession. Similarly, we become utterly convinced by and invested in the samsaric cartoon appearing before and within us. The Buddha explained that it is our inability or unwillingness to recognise the illusory nature of this self and our habitual clinging to it that lies at the root of so much of our suffering.

The problem of suffering or *Dukkha* is integral to the Buddhist teachings (Bechert and Gombrich 1998). *Dukkha* is quite a broad, encompassing term, which can include both physical and psychological suffering and distress, in addition to a more subtle yet pervading sense of unsatisfactoriness or not-quite-rightness that characterises much of daily life. One particularly relatable etymology for *Dukkha* describes a badly fitted wheel that doesn't turn properly on its axle – similar to the familiar problematic trolley at the supermarket, that despite all our best efforts, repeatedly defies our attempts to steer in a straight line, insisting on drifting always just to the side. We may also subsequently find ourselves mistakenly projecting and attributing a self onto the trolley, becoming angry with it, perhaps even cursing and shouting abuse at it for being so uncooperative.

Our frustrating experience of the faulty turning wheel of the shopping trolley is only a tiny part of life on the larger, samsaric wheel. Although seemingly static in the iconography, the Wheel of Life turns in perpetuity, fuelled by ignorance, hatred and craving – symbolised at the centre of the wheel by the image of a pig, a snake and a rooster, respectively. Outside this centre lie several concentric circles each containing various realms of existence and experience.

Our attention is more typically drawn to the colourful activity around the centre of the wheel, where we see depicted the six domains of desire. These realms include the heavens, the realm of the demi-gods, human and animal realms, followed by the more disturbing hells and the realm of the hungry ghosts. Each of these realms has its psychological counterpart, the heat of rage and hatred is the hell realm, the mental state of craving and addiction is represented by the hungry ghosts, and states of great bliss and enjoyment may be reflected in the heavenly realm.

In the top left-hand corner of this particular Tibetan painting (Figure 3.1), beyond the wheel of life, within the stylised clouds, one can see the 'Pure Land' of the Buddha of infinite light, *Amitabha*. One might reasonably ask *where* or *what* is the Pure Land? The Buddhist nun I Tsao Fashih explains that it is as much a state of mind as it is celestial realm:

> The Pure Land is called the highest happiness . . .
>
> When I walk I am stepping on lotus flowers, so I am always happy. When I pass away I will go to the Pure Land; however, I realize that right now too I am living in the Pure Land.
>
> *(Batchelor 1998, pp. 68–69)*

The psychological dimension of these realms is also emphasised in the popular Japanese tale of the Samurai who challenged a Zen master to explain to him the nature of heaven and hell. Instead of answering his question, the Zen master cruelly insults him. The Samurai is utterly humiliated and draws his sword in ferocious anger – fully intending to decapitate the master. With a piercing shout, the Zen master declares, 'Here are the gates of hell!' At that very moment, the Samurai sees his own terrifying reflection within the blade of his sword – his eyes bloodshot, his face red with rage, his jaw clenched into a grimace – appearing just like a denizen of the hell realms. Overcome with shock, shame and gratitude for this teaching, the Samurai lowers his sword and bows in apology. Observing his sincere contrition and new-found humility, the Zen Master remarks, 'Here are the gates of heaven.'

These sorts of stories suggest that the distance and difference between hell and heaven and between ordinary perception and the Pure Land may be traversed or transformed by a single awakened thought or feeling.

Only the human realm affords us the opportunity to awaken and leave the wheel of life. For this reason, it is often referred to as the precious human birth in Tibetan Buddhist teachings. In this realm, we are understood to be neither excessively tormented by suffering nor too blinded by bliss to seek emancipation.

Seeing Clearly and Looking Beyond

If one's attention moves to the lesser studied, outer rim of the wheel of life, one will notice some illustrations which depict the twelve links of dependent origination or *Paṭiccasamuppāda*. This rather complex sequence describes how consciousness comes to be and operates, from life to life and moment to moment. The process begins with and in ignorance, before progressing to mental formations, consciousness, name and form, the six senses (including the mind), contact, feeling, desire, clinging, becoming, and birth leading to old age and death (Bechert and Gombrich 1998).

If one can see and understand this process, then one is said to see the core of the Buddha's teaching, or Dharma. These links describe how we remain chained within the Samsaric cycle.

Our contact with the world, mediated through our senses, habitually leads to our being attracted or repulsed by what we encounter. These attractions and repulsions feed into various fixations and cravings for and clinging to more of what we desire and less of what don't desire. Through this process, we are repeatedly and unconsciously pulled along paths that lead directly to suffering.

We have become so habituated to these processes that we barely notice them, and their links follow in such rapid succession that contact with an object and our conditioned reaction to it is experienced as instantaneous. It all seems to happen of its own accord. In this way, it is not too dissimilar from Freud's original conception of the unconscious as *Das Es*, 'the it' (Bettelheim 2001) – as in 'I didn't mean to react that way, speak those hurtful words or break that plate in a fit of rage – *it* just happened!' Behaviourists would likely describe this process as being due to conditioning and repeated reinforcement. Cognitive Psychologists may prefer to describe this process as being the result of automaticity – but the key, defining factor remains, that it occurs either without or before our conscious awareness.

Through meditation one endeavours to disrupt the links of dependent origination and in so doing escape the *samsaric* cycle. The key to doing this, but not the shortcut, is slowing down.

The key requires retraining ourselves to notice the very moment that attraction or repulsion arises. In the twelve links of dependent origination, this moment occurs immediately after, seemingly simultaneously with the moment of contact with an object, and is named *vedanā* – feeling (Peacock and Batchelor 2020). *Vedanā* refers to the feelings of attraction or repulsion, our habitual reactivity towards whatever one is seeing, hearing, touching, tasting or experiencing. Through cultivating mindfulness of *vedanā*, one may disrupt, reverse and escape the cycle, but one must first effectively slow the cycle, in order to clearly see it in action. In meditation, one is effectively learning to perceive the thoughts and feelings with far greater clarity, with the intention of being able to *respond* to them creatively rather than *reacting* habitually.

Looking and seeing clearly becomes a relatable, tangible way of describing the Buddhist process of awakening. It is significant that in the Buddha's Noble Eightfold Path, the very first attainment is *Sammādiṭṭhi* – realising the Right View. As Paul Swanson, a leading scholar of the Chinese Buddhist *Tian Tai* tradition, reflects,

> the purpose of Buddhism is clarity; it is the search for clarity. To feel clearly, so as to avoid damaging passions; to see clearly, so as to be able to respond to circumstances in a positive and healthy way; to think clearly, so as to act with wisdom and compassion.
>
> *(Swanson 2018, p. 1)*

Buddhist Psychology

In addition to the recorded teachings of the Buddha found in the Buddhist scriptures, the various collections of *Sutras*, one also finds the lesser-known *Abhidhamma* tradition and texts which painstakingly observe, record and contrast the varied and complex states and stages of deluded perception, thought and feeling, precisely guiding one towards more awakened states and stages. For example, one frequently used term found throughout a great many Buddhist texts and teachings is *citta*, more commonly referring to one's heart and mind, a concept which becomes far more complex and multifaceted in *Abdhidhamma*. Jacobs (2017) describes the Abhidhamma as 'The Original Buddhist Psychology', but her description of *cittas* appears to extend into the realm of physics:

> Cittas can perform many functions within the realm of basic knowing and also have various important qualities in the Abhidharma system. They can operate in more concrete or subtle spheres, they can be associated with different subqualities (like different electron formations around a proton), and they can have different relationships in the realm of causality. They are categorised according to all of this into either 89 or 121 types, depending on how you count certain cognitive functions that only apply to the most adept meditators and enlightened people.
>
> *(Ibid., p. 21)*

One of the earliest scholars to refer explicitly to 'Buddhist Psychology' was the celebrated translator of the Pali Canon and former President of the British Pali Text Society (1923–1942), Caroline Rhys Davids, whose own analysis of the *Abdhidhamma* led to her praising the 'introspective genius of Buddhism'

(Rhys Davids 2018, pp. v–vi), which she had hoped the newly emerging field of Psychology would attend to in order to learn from and build upon.

It is however worth noting that these texts are usually the preserve of scholastic monks, academics and Buddhist specialists. It is also equally important to note that the primary purpose and function of *Abhidhamma* is soteriological rather than psychological – that is to say that they are far less concerned with achieving a passive, theoretical account of cognition and affect, and are far more focused on actively transforming, awakening and liberating our consciousness from the wheel of life.

The teachings of the Buddha, known collectively as the *Buddhadharma*, are also commonly symbolised with a wheel. The various teachings of the Buddha are described as the turning of the wheel of Dharma (Bechert and Gombrich 1998). The wheel of Dharma turns in a conscious countermotion to the wheel of life, effectively slowing before stopping it, thereby allowing one to exit.

In this way, the wheel of life seems akin to a karmic carnival ride, perhaps most similar to Gravitrons, found at funfairs around the world. One stands within the Gravitron, and as it turns faster and faster, the centripetal force generated by the momentum presses one's back against the carriage and one is rendered temporarily immobile. One may only look directly ahead as it becomes increasingly difficult to move. Only as the ride slows does one regain increasingly more control over one's movements, and only when it stops one can safely disembark. In most depictions of the wheel of life, one can see the Buddha standing outside of and above the wheel, gesturing towards it and the various processes keeping us firmly fixed to and held within it.

The Speed and Nature of Thought

A popular translation of the first verse of *Dhammapada* begins with a statement that typically excites and encourages psychologists and psychotherapists:

> We are what we think.
> All that we are arises with our thoughts.
> With our thoughts we make the world.
> (Kornfield 1996, p. 4)

This verse is sometimes presented as the Buddhist equivalent to the Bible's iconic opening 'In the Beginning', although in this instance, the beginning is not referring to the origin of the world or an act of a creation via a creator God but rather the content of our own minds. This more secular sounding statement also leads to the very popular, contemporary contention in the West that Buddhism is far less of a religion in the familiar mould of centring around adherence to doctrine or requiring faith, and much more of an empirical 'mind science' – a term which the current Dalai Lama et al. (2012) remain particularly fond of.

The first *Dhammapada* verse, when translated in this manner, appears to be advocating a particular form of idealism, more commonly encountered in the later *Yogācāra* school of Buddhism, alternately known by the name *citta-mātra* meaning 'mind only' school (Tagawa 2009). According to some interpretations of *Yogācāra*, the physical world may be understood as a mere projection of one's own mind – my thoughts are not just things, things are just my thoughts – and subsequently 'with our thoughts we make the world'.

A more technically accurate translation renders this same verse:

> Fore-run by mind are mental states,
> Ruled by mind, made of mind.
> (Roebuck 2010, p. 3)

Here the scope of mind appears significantly narrowed, pertaining specifically to our mental states. The verse proceeds to note the inevitable karmic consequences of unwholesome thoughts, words and deeds:

> If you speak or act
> With corrupt mind,
> Suffering follows you,
> As the wheel the foot of the ox.
> (Ibid., p. 3)

In this early scripture, we are first introduced to the comparison of the mind with an ox pulling the wheel of a cart, and we are subsequently enjoined to guide our minds into more stable states of clarity which brings joy and allows for a smoother journey through life. One may also further reflect on whether we are yoking ourselves to the Samsaric wheel of life or the wheel of Dharma.

In a related popular allegory of the Chinese Chan, the Japanese Zen and the Korean Sŏn schools of Buddhism, the ox reappears in the 'Ten Ox-Herding' pictures. These pictures are intended to illustrate the practice of meditation, through ten stages of the contemplative path and practice – beginning with one's setting out and searching and ending with one's awakening and returning.

The most popular scene from this series is the sixth stage, frequently reproduced in Chinese painting and sculpture, and depicts a young boy effortlessly 'riding the ox home' whilst playing a flute. It is important to remember that this scene of ease is the result of a great deal of effort and perseverance; taken in isolation it belies the considerable psychological struggle that enabled it to take place.

The preceding pictures with their accompanying poetic verses depict the challenging, often frustrating process of meditation – the practice of finding, training, taming and even transcending the mind. Beginning with the search in earnest for the ox, the quest to encounter our mind, we see a young ox herder wandering alone through a forest in search of the ox:

> High mountains, deep waters, and a dense jungle of grass-
> However much you try, the way to proceed remains unclear!
> (Kusan 1985, p. 153)

Beginners in meditative practice might find that the above verse reflects and resonates with their first experience of sitting. One may expect meditation to make the mind calm and tranquil, but in stark contrast the first experience many newcomers have is how loud and disorientating their ordinary mind is – it is quite easy to get lost in the endless chatter and clamour of our thoughts.

How might one use the mind to tame the mind? How does one become aware of awareness itself? With persistent, patient practice, we begin to perceive and follow the footprints of the ox in the second stage and verse – we see where the mind has previously been through refining our powers of reflection and recollection.

Eventually, in the third stage, we may catch our first fleeting glimpse of the ox itself. Typically, we see the tail of the ox first (Kusan 1985, p. 158), just as we may notice the tail end of a passing thought or feeling and realise that the mind is wandering, before we return and redirect our attention back to the practice. With time and effort, the ox becomes clearer, more present and defined, allowing us to try and catch the ox in the fourth stage. Yet catching the ox is no easy endeavour, as our attempts to pierce the nose and rein it in may frequently be foiled as we are dragged along by the powerful beast, or else repeatedly losing it in the jungle as it swiftly evades us. The ox is clearly craftier and far faster than we thought.

But just how fast is a thought? We are confidently informed by physicists that nothing can exceed the speed of light – which is calculated as 186,000 miles per second. If we accept a materialist world view that argues consciousness is a particular type of epiphenomenon, a by-product of organic brain function, explained and understood as emerging from the firing of neurons, registering as electrochemical signals – then thought is just another category of thing, consisting of physical properties, contained within and constrained by the same physical laws that govern the rest of the universe.

In the *Yogācāra* school of Buddhism, they sought to quantify the speed of thought through their identification and analysis of the *cittakṣaṇa* – the thought moment. This moment was so infinitesimal as to be almost imperceptible:

> Dogen Zenji said that most people are not able to acquire the way-seeking mind of spiritual awareness without deeply understanding that a day consists of 6,400,099,180 moments.
>
> . . . A moment is called ksana in Sanskrit. Sometimes we say that one finger snap has sixty moments, so one finger snap equals sixty ksana. A Buddhist dictionary may say that a moment equals one seventy-fifth of a second. According to the Abhidharma scriptures, a moment consists of sixty-five instants.
>
> *(Katagiri 2007, p. 3)*

Such reflections lead one to a challenging and disconcerting question – How are we to achieve any authentic awareness or transformation of our own minds, if our world and thoughts travel so fast?

And speed is far from the only obstacle preventing our achieving 'the way-seeking mind of spiritual awareness' (Ibid.). Our age is defined by distractions. Our assortment of digital devices may be quite accurately characterised as 'weapons of mass distraction'. In the digital age of multitasking, it is not unusual to find ourselves watching a film, whilst also browsing online and texting a friend, whilst simultaneously chatting to the person sitting right next to us. We now have distractions to distract us from our distractions.

Our attention spans may feel as though they are getting shorter, whilst our attention itself is increasingly, chronically divided. What Buddhists refer to as the *citta-saṃtāna* – mind stream, or the Jamesian stream of consciousness – is more swiftly coming to resemble a series of tumultuous torrents and rapidly flowing rivulets.

Citta Slow – Stilling Heart and Mind

When I first heard of the Cittaslow movement, I had incorrectly assumed that it was a Buddhist-inspired, mindfulness-based movement – as *citta* in Sanskrit refers to both the heart and mind. I was very already very familiar with Mahayana Buddhist Sanskrit terms such as *Bodhicitta* – the awakened heart-mind of an aspiring Buddha, exemplified by a being who is suffused with selfless compassion and loving-kindness. In the case of the Cittaslow movement, *città* is the Italian word for city, yet I maintain that a Buddhist reading of the term reveals something of the heart essence of meditative practice.

Almost all Buddhist practice and mindfulness-based approaches encourage and instruct us in how to '*citta* slow' – to steady the racing pace of our thoughts. Mindfulness is synonymous with slow living – indeed it is its very foundation.

Contemporary mindfulness practices can usually trace their roots back to the original Buddhist meditative traditions of *Samatha* and *Vipassana*.

Samatha refers to the process of calming, settling and stilling the mind into a tranquil, focused and flexible state. *Vipassana*, which translates to enhanced seeing, refers to this settled mind's penetrating insight into and realisation of the unsatisfactory, impermanent and ultimately selfless nature of reality.

As *Samatha* is usually the first practice a beginner might encounter, this may lead to the misnomer that *Samatha* is *only* a beginner's practice. This view often overlooks *Samatha* as a demanding, comprehensive and graduated practice.

Samatha and *Vipassana* remained the central practices of the earliest native school of Chinese Buddhism, the ancestor of Zen Buddhism, the *Tian Tai* school. The Chinese term for *Samatha* is *Zhi* 止, which refers to stopping, whereas Vipassana is *Guan* 觀, which refers to seeing. So, in the Chinese Buddhist tradition, *Samatha* and *Vipassana* are equivalent to the contemplative practice and process of stopping in order to clearly observe the contents of one's mind.

It is often argued, particularly when taught in contemporary Western contexts, that 'stopping' does not and should not refer to a literal stopping of thoughts but rather the stopping of distractions and mental afflictions leading to greater clarity, and clearer observation of one's thoughts. The standard advice provided by modern teachers of mindfulness emphasises that practitioners should *not* be trying to suppress their thoughts or silence their minds. Whilst I would agree that for a beginner any forceful, artificially imposed attempts to quell the chatter in their minds would likely be counterproductive, more advanced practitioners *have* consciously sought out and reported meditative realms where the practitioner experiences a complete cessation of thought – these are mental realms, unchartered depths that mainstream psychology appears neither equipped nor inclined to explore further, and yet according to many Buddhist schools these transcendent states bring us closer to our original mind or Buddha Nature.

This stopping or stilling element is beautifully expressed in the Tibetan Buddhist *Dzogchen* teachings, where one encounters *Samatha*-style, pith instructions, as one of my former Tibetan teachers explained with this poetic aphorism:

ཆུ་མ་རྙོག་ན་དྭངས། སེམས་མ་བཅོས་ན་བདེ།
Chu ma nyok na dang. Sem ma chö na dé
Water, when undisturbed, is clear. Mind, when uncontrived, is at ease.

An accompanying visual example may be of the familiar school science experiment where a transparent glass beaker filled with dark, opaque water, clouded with sediment is simply left untouched and unstirred for up to an hour. Over time, the sediment settles and sinks to the bottom of the beaker and the water becomes clear. Likewise, if one can learn to stop stirring and disturbing the mind with rancorous or anxious rumination and destructive emotions, a natural clarity and inherent purity returns.

Water-related imagery is quite commonly found on mindfulness promotional materials, books and websites including serene scenes of tranquil pools of water, sometimes adorned with stacked stones or rising lotus flowers. A very popular metaphor used by traditional Buddhist meditation masters and secular mindfulness teachers alike in relation to clearly seeing is to consider one's state of mind as if one were gazing into a pool of water. When the surface of the water is disturbed, one can perceive only the ripples, bubbles and froth – the thoughts, feelings and sensations. However, when the surface is calm, one begins to see one's face clearly reflected and also, eventually what lies beneath.

What lies beneath or beyond is arguably of less interest to more secular-minded psychotherapists, whose primary interests and priorities concern treating anxiety states and depressive episodes. Most mindfulness-based approaches tend to limit themselves to enhancing the metacognitive capacities of their clients – being able to think *about* their thoughts and able to challenge their negative automatic thoughts (NATs). By contrast, traditional *Samatha* practice and *Abhidhammic* texts extend far beyond our ordinary, everyday thoughts and feelings into transcognitive and transpersonal realms.

The Buddhist monk Bhante Henepola Gunaratana has been particularly keen to promote the deeper states of prolonged *Samatha* practice in 'Beyond Mindfulness in Plain English' (Gunaratana 2009). These deeper states of meditation are referred to in Buddhist texts as the *Jhānas* – profound states of meditative absorption and concentration (Nyanatiloka 1997, pp. 83–85), a stillness and serenity which progresses beyond all thoughts, feelings and sensations of the perceptual realm. The *Jhanas* themselves are divided into eight types; four material and four immaterial states. The progression through the first two material *Jhānas* already appears to be approaching a more literal stopping and cessation of one's thoughts:

> The world goes away. Physical pain goes away. You do not totally lose all sensation, but the physical senses are all off in the background. Wandering conscious thoughts stop. What remains are subtle thoughts of good will towards all beings.
>
> *(Gunaratana 2009, pp. 104–105)*

And by the second Jhana:

> The subtle thoughts of good will drop away. Your mind is now totally free of any verbal or conceptual thoughts, even that of the breath.
>
> *(Ibid., p. 105)*

Having already ventured well beyond the traditional, disciplinary scope of mainstream psychology and psychotherapy, the *Jhānas* continue to progress further into two additional material states and four further immaterial states, each with increasingly esoteric-sounding designations such as the base of 'infinite space', 'infinite awareness', 'nothingness' and 'neither perception nor non-perception' (Ibid., pp. 107–108). Take a moment to consider just how far stillness can take you.

To successfully cultivate such advanced meditative states takes time and patience. Both Samatha and Vipassana are understood by Buddhist meditators as lifelong practices, an attitude and approach that appear wholly at odds with our shortcut culture. Meditation aids such as Holosync®, marketed as a 'brainwave stimulator', claim to enable one to 'Meditate 8x faster than a Zen monk at the touch of a button' (a claim I evaluate further in Chapter 6).

In the race towards awakening, *Samatha* practice is frequently overlooked for practices that are perceived as being more challenging, advanced or intriguing. Popular examples might include endurance style Zen practices of *Shikantaza* 'Just Sitting', or meditation using a *Koan* – a statement intended to invite reflection, exhaust and transcend the intellect, leading to a direct experience of awakening – 'What is the sound of one hand clapping?' or the equally cryptic 'What is this?' For those seeking something even more exotic and esoteric, they might attempt highly demanding Tibetan visualisation techniques involving complex, colourful, three-dimensional mandalas. An esteemed Western teacher of *Samatha* meditation and author of 'The Attention Revolution', B. Alan Wallace (2006), voices frustration regarding contemporary contemplative trends:

> Hardly anyone heeds the counsel of the great meditators of Tibet's past who claim the achievement of Shamatha is necessary for all advanced forms of meditation to be fully effective. A mind easily distracted or prone to dullness is simply unfit for meditation of any kind.
>
> I find it astonishing that the training of attention has been so marginalized both in modern science and in many contemplative traditions.
>
> *(Ibid., p. xii)*

I do not personally share Wallace's astonishment however, as I believe that due to our velocentric lifestyles, we are psychologically predisposed to seek shortcuts over disciplined practice and stimulation over stillness.

Seeing Beyond the Waves and Remembering the Mountain

In order to demonstrate our habitual preference for stimulation over stillness, we might consider the famous woodblock print 'Under the Great Wave of Kanagawa' by the renowned Japanese Buddhist artist Katsushika Hokusai (1760–1849). 'The Great Wave' (see Figure 3.2), as it is often known, was and remains one of the most reproduced images in the history of art and has become a familiar staple of pop culture. Sometimes in class, I ask my students to simply say what they see – the first answers are not surprisingly 'a great tidal wave' or 'fishing boats'. When one looks at the print, one's attention is typically, automatically drawn towards the great towering waves, rising ominously high over the fishing boats, moments before we imagine they are about to crash down upon the poor, unfortunate fishermen. One may reflect upon the awesome, unbridled, raw power of nature, depicted in the waves, and the comparative fragility and vulnerability of the human world represented by the fishing boats. One can easily lose oneself in the action and ensuing chaos of the scene, and yet near the centre of the print, rising from the sea, almost to be mistaken as another wave, is a still, calm counterpoint – Mount Fuji.

Fuji sits serenely in the background of this scene, like the eye of a hurricane. It is important to remember that despite its iconic status, 'The Great Wave' was only one in a series titled 'Thirty-Six Views of Mount Fuji' (Guth 2016). It is also worth noting that Fuji is much more than a mere mountain in Japanese culture and is considered to be the sacred residing place of the Goddess *Konohanasakuya-hime*. An ambivalent nature deity, *Konohanasakuya-hime*

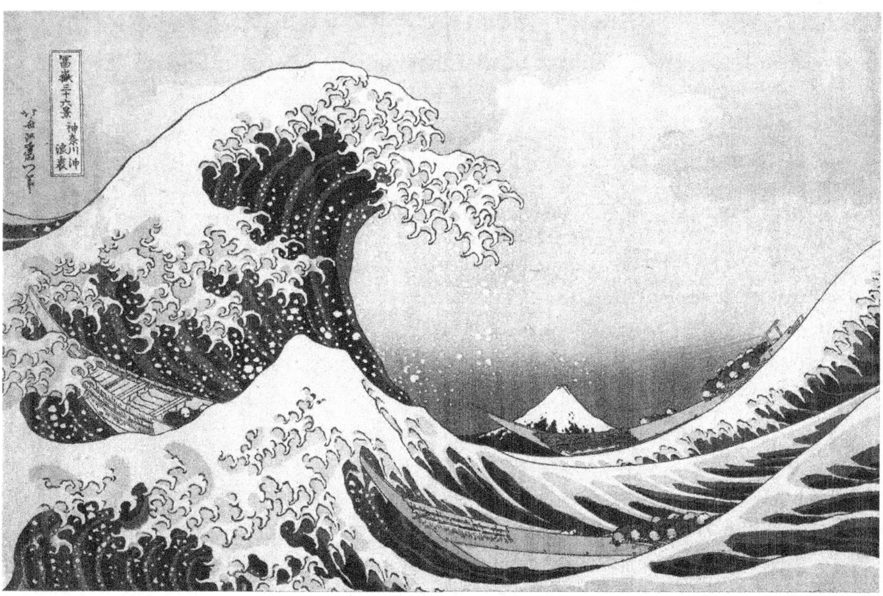

FIGURE 3.2 The Great Wave off Kanagawa' by Hokusai

combines apparent contradictions – in addition to being the Goddess of volcanoes, with their characteristic fire, fury and destructive capacity, She is also a Goddess of life and nature whose symbol is the delicate, fragile Cherry blossom.

When viewing Hokusai's famous print, we first see and are seduced by the crashing waves and can easily forget or fail to notice the still, divine mountain. In this way, it may help to view 'The Great Wave' through the lens of the *Mundaka Upanishad*, and to compare the frenetic activity of the waves with the busy bird seeking the pipala fruits, whilst the still, silent, witnessing bird sat at the top of the tree may be related to the abiding, anchoring presence of Mount Fuji.

Hokusai is arguably the best-known representative of a Japanese artistic genre known as *Ukiyo-e* 浮き世, which translates into the poetic and evocative term 'Pictures of the Floating World' (Davis 2021). This term has its roots in Buddhism and teachings related to *Anicca* – the impermanence of all conditioned reality. The original Japanese characters for *Ukiyo* 憂き世 referred to the sorrowful samsaric realm, but this was later changed into a more playful pun as the first character was replaced with *uki* 浮, referring to floating. *Ukiyo-e* prints often include themes depicting both the beauty and the ephemera of the natural world, celebrating both the ordinariness and momentariness of human life. A frequent theme found in *Ukiyo-e* includes the marking of the seasons, particularly the quintessential *Sakura* Cherry Blossom festivals still observed around Japan. The delicate, pink showers of cherry blossom raining down with each gust of wind evoke a strong national appreciation for impermanence, visually conveying both the beauty and poignancy of life. Whereas traditionally *Anicca* is directly related to *Dukkha*, in Japanese aesthetics, shaped and informed by Zen Buddhism, one seeks and appreciates the beauty and preciousness endowed by impermanence. The uniqueness of each person, each flower, each moment and motion, is expressed in the Japanese phrase *ichi-go ichi-e* 一期一会 which translates to 'one time, one meeting', a phrase and philosophy popularly attributed to the great sixteenth-century Zen tea master Sen No Rikyū (Varley and Kumakura 1989). *Ichi-go ichi-e* reminds one to endeavour to treasure each and every one of life's varied encounters. Rikyū is widely celebrated and acknowledged as one of the founders of the Japanese Zen tea ceremony, which itself is arguably the rightful ancestor of all modern mindful eating and drinking practices.

Drinking Tea Mindfully

One of the most influential promoters of mindfulness meditation in the West was the Vietnamese Zen Buddhist monk Thich Nhat Hanh (1926–2022). Nhat Hanh's consistent emphasis on mindfulness was intended to serve as a much-needed alternative to our dromocratic cultures of chronic distraction and dissatisfaction, as such he was an ardent advocate of slow living:

> People today do not know how to rest. They fill their free time with countless diversions. People cannot tolerate even a few minutes of unoccupied time. They have to turn on the TV or pick up a newspaper, reading anything at all, even the advertisements. They constantly need something to look at, listen to, or talk about, all to keep the emptiness inside from rearing its terrifying head.
>
> *(Nhat Hanh 2001, p. 45)*

In introducing his students to mindfulness, Nhat Hanh would typically take familiar and often mundane daily activities, sweeping the yard or washing the dishes, and demonstrate how we might make the familiar strange, the ordinary extraordinary, simply by slowing down and noticing more. One example might be the tea ceremonies that took place at Nhat Hanh's monastery at Plum Village in Loubès-Bernac, France.

Tea frequently plays a central role in Zen Buddhism. England is also a tea culture. Tea remains the iconic national drink, but the manner in which it is typically drunk differs greatly from the more ceremonial styles of Chinese and Japanese culture. In England, we *have* a cup of tea – its actual place in our social interactions is arguably quite peripheral, and its primary purpose is more divertive – to soothe and serve as social lubricant, and often to encourage and facilitate conversation (Cohen 2009).

In Chinese and Japanese tea ceremonies, there is more a sense of *being* with a cup of tea. The various forms of Zen tea ritual emerged from and embody many core principles of Buddhist practice and are also examples par excellence of slow living, slow food, slow eating and drinking.

Tea was traditionally used to refresh the monks between long periods of sitting practice, but soon became integrated into the meditative practice, developing into various tea-centred rituals. Despite its beginnings in China, the Zen tea ceremonies of Japan are perhaps the best known for their slow, precise movements and immersive, aesthetic appeal.

The tea ceremonies constitute some of the earliest examples of mindful eating and drinking practices. Mindful eating practices, particularly 'raisin exercise' (Didonna 2009) has become a very popular way of introducing mindfulness to beginners. The exercise works by taking a seemingly unremarkable activity such as eating a small, single raisin, and demonstrates how, by intentionally slowing, holding, looking, smelling and tasting more deeply, as opposed to mindlessly scoffing, the experience becomes far more engaging and enriching, even moving.

The purpose of these practices is to transform our ordinary, more automatic ways of drinking into a more conscious consuming. Every element of the tea drinking, including its preparation, becomes central:

> Prepare a pot of tea to serve a guest or to drink by yourself. Do each movement slowly, in mindfulness. Do not let one detail of your movements go by without being mindful of it. Know that your hand lifts the pot by its handle. Know that you are pouring the fragrant warm tea into the cup. Follow each step in mindfulness. Breathe gently and more deeply than usual. Take hold of your breath if your mind strays.
>
> *(Nhat Hanh 1991, p. 85)*

The drinking of tea became an extension of Zen sitting practice. Well-known Chinese Buddhist expressions such as *Cha Chan Yi Wei* 茶禪一味, Tea and Zen are of One Taste, encapsulate this sentiment. That drinking tea with *Cha Xin*, 茶心, tea-mind is equivalent to *Chan* 禪 (Zen), a Chinese term originally used to refer to deep meditative states of *Jhana* cultivated during *Samatha* meditation.

The Great Taiwanese Buddhist master Hsing Yun goes further to equate the simple experience of drinking tea with awakening itself:

> What is the Way? What is awakening? They are the same as drinking tea. The mind may tell you it is something different, but one should not depart from everyday life. It is within everyday life that one finds the Way.
>
> *(Hsing Yun 2018, p. 9)*

Drinking tea is transformed into a meditative act through deliberately slowing. The simple act of slowing imbues and empowers one's actions with a profound sense of ceremony and significance. Tea becomes more than a mere beverage, but a way – *Cha Dao* 茶道 the way of tea.

One of the earliest and most popular Chinese poems in praise of tea, titled 'Seven Bowls of Tea', was composed by Lu Tong (790–835) in the Tang Dynasty. This short poem extols the spiritual value of tea and its capacity to allow us to taste the transcendent. In a manner which appears to parallel and progress through Maslow's familiar hierarchy of needs and beyond to the 'Farther Reaches of Human Nature' (Maslow 1993). It begins with the physiological need for sustenance and refreshment:

> The first bowl moistens my lips and throat.
>
> *(Lu Tong quoted in Benn 2015, p. 14)*

The subsequent needs of safety and belonging appear to be addressed in the following line:

> The second bowl banishes my loneliness and melancholy.
>
> *(Ibid.)*

The final lines express transcendence and have an unmistakably transpersonal tone:

> The sixth bowl allows me to communicate with the immortals.
> The seventh bowl I need not drink,
> I am aware of a pure wind rising beneath my two arms.
> The Mountains of Penglai, what is this place?
> I, Master of the Jade Stream, ride this pure wind and wish to return home.
>
> (Ibid., p. 15)

The Penglai that Lu Tong refers to is a legendary land of immortal beings, popular in Daoist lore, quite similar to the Pure Lands described in Mahayana Buddhism.

When we allow the mind to rest and the thoughts to still, settle and sink, like tea leaves to the bottom of the bowl, one's seeing and one's very being become infused with greater clarity. If, as the Dhammapada described, our thoughts do indeed make our world, then perhaps the way to Penglai is merely a matter of calming our restless minds and purifying our perception.

References

Batchelor, M. (1998) *Walking on Lotus Flowers: Buddhist Women Living, Loving and Meditating*. London: Thorsons.

Bechert, H. and Gombrich, R. (1998) *The World of Buddhism*. London: Thames and Hudson.

Benn, J. A. (2015) *Tea in China: A Religious and Cultural History*. Honolulu, HI: University of Hawaii Press.

Bettelheim, B. (2001) *Freud and Man's Soul*. London: Pimlico.

Cohen, E. (2009) A tantalising taste of the timeless transcendent: An adaptation of the Zen Tea ceremony for use with enhanced care service users within the National Health Service. *Transpersonal Psychology Review*, 13(1), pp. 29–37.

Dalai Lama, L., Benson, H., Thurman, R., Gardner, H. and Goleman, D. (2012) *MindScience: An East West Dialogue*. New York: Wisdom Publications.

Davis, J. N. (2021) *Picturing the Floating World: Ukiyo-e in Context*. Honolulu, HI: University of Hawai'i Press.

Didonna, F. (Ed.) (2009) *Clinical Handbook of Mindfulness*. New York: Springer.

Gunaratana, H. (2009) *Beyond Mindfulness in Plain English*. Boston, MA: Shambhala Publications.

Guth, C. (2016) *Hokusai's Great Wave: Biography of a Global Icon*. Honolulu, HI: University of Hawai'i Press.

Hsing Yun (2018) *Buddhism and the Tea Ceremony*. Kaohsiung: Fo Guang Shan International Translation Centre.

Jacobs, B. (2017) *The Original Buddhist Psychology*. Berkeley, CA: North Atlantic Books.

Katagiri, D. (2007) *Each Moment Is the Universe: Zen and the Way of Being Time*. Boston, MA: Shambhala.

Kornfield, J. (1996) *Teachings of the Buddha*. Boston, MA: Shambhala Publications.

Kusan, S. (1985) *The Way of Korean Zen*. Boston, MA: Weatherhill.

Maslow, A. (1993) *The Farther Reaches of Human Nature*. New York: Penguin Arkana.

Nhat Hanh, T. (1991) *The Miracle of Mindfulness*. New York: Rider.
Nhat Hanh, T. (2001) *Thich Nhat Hanh: Essential Writings*. New York: Orbis Books.
Nyanatiloka, V. (1997) *Buddhist Dictionary: Manual of Buddhist Terms and Doctrines*. Kandy: Buddhist Publication Society.
Peacock, J. and Batchelor, M. (2020) *The Definition, Practice and Psychology of Vedanā: Knowing How It Feels*. Oxon: Routledge.
Rhys Davids, C. (2018) *Buddhist Psychology: An Inquiry into the Analysis and Theory of Mind in Pali Literature*. London: Forgotten Books.
Roebuck, V. (Trans.) (2010) *The Dhammapada*. London: Penguin Books.
Swanson, P. L. (2018) *In Search of Clarity: Essays on Translation and Tiantai Buddhism*. Nagoya: Chisokudō Publications.
Tagawa, S. (2009) *Living Yogācāra: An Introduction to Consciousness-Only Buddhism*. Boston, MA: Wisdom Publications.
Varley, P. and Kumakura, I. (Eds.) (1989) *Tea in Japan: Essays on the History of Chanoyu*. Honolulu, HI: University of Hawai'i Press.
Wallace, B. A. (2006) *The Attention Revolution: Unlocking the Power of the Focused Mind*. Somerville, MA: Wisdom Publications.

4

THE DAO OF DECELERATION

Alongside Buddhism and Confucianism, Daoism has played a significant role in shaping the Chinese psyche. Indeed, a popular saying suggests that the Chinese people whilst Confucian in public are Daoist in private (Peng et al. 2006, p. 249). Some additional context may be needed to fully understand this saying – Confucianism is commonly associated with preserving traditional values and order, deference towards one's elders and betters, whereas Daoism is perceived as being more individualistic, emphasising qualities of ease and spontaneity. To cautiously apply a well-known Western, Nietzschean comparative framework, we might say that Confucianism is more Apollonian, whilst Daoism is more Dionysian.

Confucians praise those who chisel and polish the jade – referring to those who tirelessly work upon themselves, correcting, realigning their character and refining their nature. Daoists admire the stone in its original state – uncarved, uncontrived and unadorned. In practice, it requires just as much effort to carve the stone as it does to return to an uncarved block following a lifetime of socialisation and cultural conditioning. To be Confucian in public suggests that one carefully maintains the appearance of obedience, bound by the bonds of family and community, whilst in private one remains unbound and free to express oneself in the manner one wishes. It is not entirely clear whether 'private' in this instance refers to one's own home or the free domain of the mind, but implicitly the saying seems to suggest that Daoism allows for a more intimate, non-contrived encounter.

Daoism is an indigenous, at once ancient and living Chinese tradition that includes, but eludes any essentialist reduction to, religion, philosophy, physiology, psychology, ecology and various cultivations arts and practices

DOI: 10.4324/9781003334972-4

centred around healing, physical, psychological transformation and spiritual transcendence.

Definitively defining Daoism (or Taoism in its earlier forms of transliteration) is inherently challenging and often frustrating, as demonstrated in one of the most popular translations of the first verse of the seminal Daoist scripture the *Dao De Jing*:

> The Tao that can be told is not the eternal Tao.
> The name that can be named is not the eternal name.
> The nameless is the beginning of heaven and earth.
> (Feng and English 1996)

Whilst being one of the best known, frequently translated and quoted East Asian religious scriptures, it is also one of the few scriptures that begins by warning us not to become too reliant on religious utterances, even those found within scriptures.

Dao 道 is translated as the 'Way' or 'Path' – but the way to what or the path to where? I would propose that seeking and cultivating the Dao is ultimately intended to lead us back to authenticity (Kohn 2011) – a profound, transformational sense of connectedness and wholeness. Daoism traditionally sought and continues to seek to recover a deep inherent harmony between Heaven, Earth and Humanity. A fundamental principle of Daoist teachings is that human nature is *a part of* not *apart from* the natural world and order – this core principle has paradigm-shifting implications for both Psychology and Ecology.

From a Daoist perspective, humanity has become mired in artificiality, a disaffected assemblage of increasingly synthetic selves growing ever more distant and alienated from one another and from our natural world. Our contemporary Psychologies reflect and unwittingly reproduce this fractured reality without the necessary means to repair it. From this perspective, popular appeals to enhancing 'well-being' or 'resilience', including therapies lightly seasoned with a more mindful Buddhist or flow-focused Daoist flavour will simply not suffice. What is required is something more revolutionary, as the Transpersonal Psychologist John Welwood explained:

> The Psychologising of Eastern contemplative disciplines – unless it is preceded by a thorough revolution in Western Psychology itself – could rob these disciplines of their spiritual substance. It could pervert them into Western mental health gimmicks and thereby prevent them from introducing the sharply alternative vision of life they are capable of bringing to us.
>
> *(John Welwood 1979, p. 181)*

It was precisely such a revolution that Abraham Maslow had sought to ferment within Psychology – proposing a more 'Taoistic' approach to the sciences:

> Clearly we as scientists, not to mention physicians, teachers or even parents, must shift our image over to a more Taoistic one. This is the one word that I can think of that summarizes succinctly the many elements of the image of a more humanistic scientist. Taoistic means asking rather than telling. It means non-intruding, non-controlling. It stresses non-interfering observation rather than a controlling manipulation. It is receptive and passive rather than active and forceful.
>
> *(Maslow 1993, p. 14)*

But such an ambitious paradigm shift would prove difficult to achieve, and Maslow tragically passed away too soon after he had begun to realise and outline his vision for a more Transpersonal and Taoistic Psychology.

Excess and Exhaustion

How do we know when enough is enough? At this point, it would be appropriate to briefly revisit the topic of slow food and consider the theme of excess through a more psychological and contemplative lens.

The study and practice of dietetics, the careful consideration of both the type and quality and quantity of food we consume, play a significant but lesser-studied role in Daoist cultivation (Kohn 2010). One might further reflect on the inauthenticity of the ingredients we consume, in our age of ultra-processed foods. One of the particular challenges of ultra-processed foods and our excessive consumption of them is that they still leave us feeling hungry and craving more, in addition to lacking nutritional value. The primary physiological purpose of eating is to provide the body with sustenance and energy, and in traditional Chinese cosmology and medicine, the concept of energy requires the study of *qi*.

Qi 氣 is translated as energy, and also refers to one's breath and vitality. *Qi* is understood to animate and pervade the physiological, psychological and spiritual realms of being, in addition to being an inherent, primordial property of the universe. In one central Daoist scripture, named after its author Liezi, humanity is understood to have arisen due to a particular blending between the *qi* of Heaven and the *qi* of Earth (Graham 1990, p. 29). Indeed, everything that we can perceive through our senses can be understood to constitute a form or expression of *qi*.

When my wife-to-be first visited my research office at Manchester Metropolitan University, she was horrified by the chaotic, precariously piled towers of papers and books that surrounded my desk, occluding the computer and keyboard whilst also blocking out much of the natural light from the small, barred window – she took a step back and audibly exclaimed, '*Sha Qi*!' – '煞氣!' This is a term one may encounter in the study of *Feng Shui* 風水, referring to a malevolent, destructive energy emitted by clutter and disorder. I recalled at that time being in the latter stages of my PhD research and struggling to maintain the focus needed to complete the thesis. I had not, until that moment, seriously considered to what extent my material working environment, which somewhat resembled a hoarder's home, was detrimentally affecting my ability to concentrate. There was simply far too much 'stuff' blocking my desk, and this had its psychological equivalent in, or perhaps was a material manifestation of the cognitive congestion impeding my academic progress. Both *Feng Shui* and Environmental Psychology share an underlying principle that there is a clear bidirectional relationship between our psychological state and the state of our environment (both built and natural) – that as we shape and fashion our environments so, in turn, do our environments form and affect us.

In Traditional Chinese Medicine (TCM), it is understood that any excess can be detrimental to our health and well-being, including an excess of emotion leading to an internal imbalance. Sadness, anger and worry are frequently listed amongst the 'internal causes' of disease that disturb our inner psychological harmony, potentially leading to physical disease. Perhaps more surprisingly, even an excess of positive emotions, such as joy, is described as having a depleting, debilitating effect due to overstimulation of the heart (Maciocia 2015, p. 261).

When we subsequently reflect upon our respective 'cultures of excess' (Slosar 2009), the relentless stoking of desires, the loss of self-control and increasingly destructive habits of mass consumption, Daoism may appear to offer a much-needed alternative way of knowing and being.

Going with One's Gut

In a recent translation of the *Dao De Jing* (chapter 12), the belly is first introduced as a central motif of Daoist teachings and contemplative practice:

> The Five Colours blind the eye.
> The Five Tones deafen the ear.
> The Five Flavours distort the palate.
> Chasing and Hunting Madden the mind.
> Hard-to-get goods trip up the stride.
> So it is that the sage
> tends to the stomach,
> not to the eye –
> 'Discarding that over there,
> They take up this over here.'
>
> (Ziporyn 2023, p. 14)

Unlike any of the other senses (the eyes, ears, taste or even the mind), the belly alone appears to simply feel and know when it is full. Comparatively, when one considers and reflects more deeply upon our daily dietary habits, including our digital diet, our mass consumption of media, and our increasing tendencies to compulsively *binge*, these teachings become increasingly pertinent.

To truly know when one is full, to feel the satisfaction of satiation is a highly prized quality. In this sense to truly be in touch with the wisdom of the stomach, to be able to sense and 'trust one's gut', leads to a more still and stable state of *zhi zu* 知足 contentment, as opposed to the perpetual pursuit of more. The wordless, intuitive knowing of the belly is akin to knowing the Dao. More recent studies of the stomach's enteric nervous system, the so-called gut-brain connection, the relatively recent discipline of neurogastroenterology, and the proposal that the stomach itself may even constitute a 'second brain' (Gershon 2019) all provide further tantalising food for thought.

When historically considering what may be termed the anatomy of the psyche, most Western systems have tended to view and locate our soul, essence or psychological core as residing in the head or the heart. In Chinese systems, by contrast, the belly is viewed as the spiritual centre and plays a central role in Daoist cultivation, as the location of the lower *dan tian* 丹田, an energetic reservoir for the storage and circulation of *qi*.

> Wisdom is like water. It resides in the lower meditation field, the belly. The head is for thinking; the heart for willing and desiring. The belly is the place for wisdom and contemplation. We 'return' to Dao's gestating presence, from this inner womb of intuitive awareness.
>
> – *Daoist Master Zhang (quoted in Saso 2012, p. 1)*

When Carl Jung was first developing his lifelong interest in the internal alchemy of Daoism, through studying his friend, Richard Wilhelm's translation of 'The Secret of the Golden Flower', he was particularly drawn to the idea of visualising and cultivating an immortal embryo, *sheng tai* 聖胎, within one's own belly (Cohen 2011). In Daoist inner alchemical texts, one is instructed to shift the centre of one's breath from the throat and chest deeper into one's belly, practicing *tai xi* 胎息 embryonic breathing – which eventually leads to a psychological and spiritual transformation or rebirth. To 'give birth to oneself' is a fitting metaphor for Analytical Psychology's primary goal of individuation – one's inner journey towards integrating all the different and dissonant elements of our psyche into a harmonious and integrated whole.

But wholeness isn't truly whole if it includes only oneself. One is advised by the Daoist sage Zhuangzi to be and breathe deeper still by bringing our attention to and breathe from our heels. To breathe from one's heels is to connect to a more subtle, 'ancestral' breath (Wang 2011, p. 44), whilst tangibly reminding us to reconnect to the natural world. This is the way that a *zhen ren* 真人, a whole, true and authentic person, breathes according to Zhuangzi. Shifting our attention from the head and the heart to the belly and the feet, one can begin to cultivate the dual wisdom of knowing when one is full and when to walk away.

The Dao of Dropping Out

In modern China, a significant number of the younger generation appear to have finally had their fill of the hyper-competitive culture that has been forged during China's race to overtake America as the next dominant world superpower. A youth movement, perhaps more accurately described as an anti-movement, has formed that refers to itself as *tang ping* 躺平, 'Lying Flat':

> the 'Lying Flat' movement and the dispirited 'Sang culture' (internet subcultures that reflect the reduced work-ethic and a lack of self-motivation felt by young people) it represents effectively evoke nationwide youth counternarratives to an intense and fast-paced corporate and social culture in contemporary China.
>
> *(Zhang and Li 2023, p. 49)*

The official response from the Chinese Communist Party (CCP) has been unequivocally one of harsh criticism, as was bluntly expressed in the *Nanfang Daily* – 'In the face of pressure, choosing to "lie flat" is not only unjust, but shameful' (quoted in Bandurski 2021).

There are some commentators who have risen to the defence of this movement. Matthew Brooker (2021) observed that 'Lying Flat contains more than a hint of Daoism, which emphasizes harmony with nature'. Wee Kek Koon's (2021) article in the *South China Morning Post* sought to sympathetically contextualise the phenomena by evoking the memory of one of China's most admired intellectuals and poets – Tao Yuanming. Yuanming also yearned for an escape from the political intrigues and bureaucracy of the day – deeply desiring solitude and subsequently abandoning his high rank in favour of becoming a recluse and pursuing poetry.

Tao Yuanming was not merely a poet, but a poetic pioneer – one of the foremost representatives of what became the *tian yuan shi* 田園詩 fields and garden poetic movement. In one of his most famous poems, 'Returning to Live in the Country', Tao Yuanming expresses a yearning to return to the natural world:

> Young, I was always free of common feeling.
> It was in my nature to love the hills and mountains.
> Mindlessly I was caught in the dust-filled trap.
> Waking up, thirty years had gone.
> The caged bird wants the old trees and air.
>
> (Ward 2007, p. 135)

The feeling of being caged or trapped is certainly one that is shared by some of the disaffected youth of China, however, so far, those who 'lie flat' appear to possess no such poetic sensibilities or aspirations.

Lying Flat represents an escape from the relentless expectations, productivity/efficiency-focused, goals and outcomes driven agenda of the rising New China. Those resisting seek to strategically make themselves useless in order to survive societal expectations relatively unscathed. One popular online meme shared by Zhang and Li (2023. p. 61) depicts a sickle unsuccessfully attempting to harvest chives which are all uncooperatively laying horizontally, the accompanying caption reads, 'The Chives that lie flat cannot easily be cut down'. This particular meme seems to resonate with the philosophy of the Daoist sage Zhuangzi, particularly in relation to his discussion of the useless tree.

In Zhuangzi's 'Inner Chapters' (Chapter 2), we are introduced to the carpenter Shih and his apprentice, who are walking through a forest, assessing each tree, in search of the perfect wood to carve. In the course of their walk, the apprentice cannot help but notice one particularly ancient, towering oak tree, and remarks upon how exceptional the timber would be. Shih dismisses the apprentice's assessment and declares that this particular tree is 'useless' (Feng and English 2008, p. 80). Later that night the carpenter is visited by the oak tree in a dream and is consequently rebuked:

> What are you comparing me with? Are you comparing me with useful trees? There are cherry, apple, pear, orange, citron, pomelo and other fruit trees. As soon as the fruit is ripe the trees are stripped and abused. Their large branches are split, and the smaller ones torn off. Their life is bitter because of their usefulness. That is why they do not live out their natural lives but are cut off in their prime. They attract the attentions of the common world. This is so for all things. As for me, I have been trying for a long time to be useless. I was almost destroyed several times. Finally I am useless, and this is very useful to me. If I had been useful, could I ever have grown so large?
>
> *(Ibid., p. 82)*

Through this and similar stories, the reader is introduced to the wisdom of *wu yong zhi yong* 無用之用 the usefulness of uselessness. In this sense, 'uselessness' may be understood as being a defence mechanism against exploitation and eventual, inevitable exhaustion. In modern China, many young people may feel reluctant to play their part in Xi Jinping and the CCP's shared vision of what is called the 'Chinese Dream' *Zhong Guo Meng* 中國夢, the Chinese equivalent of the American dream. The Chinese dream refers to the rejuvenation and revitalisation of the Chinese nation and requires of its youth to conscientiously strive and struggle to achieve its rapid realisation. For the CCP, the youth represent their collective hopes for China's bright future and are seen as their greatest resource and asset to be effectively and efficiently managed. However, the disaffected, disillusioned youth who opt out and 'lie flat' do not wish to be seen or treated as human resources, mere cogs in the machinery of the nation-state, and are consequently embodying a posture and mentality of apathy.

Those who lie flat seemingly have no alternative aspirations or dreams, other than to be left alone; feeling trapped within a state structure they feel little affinity towards or agency within they engage in various forms of non-being – no longer possessing the will or capacity to imagine doing anything or being anywhere else. Disillusioned with the Chinese Dream but not promoting or pursuing any alternative dreams of their own.

One possible alternative to this constrictive and potentially nihilistic view may also be found in Zhuangzi's 'Butterfly Dream', in which he playfully explores and expresses the ambiguity of being:

> Once upon a time, I Chuang Tsu, dreamed I was a butterfly flying happily here and there, enjoying life without knowing who I was. Suddenly I woke up and I was indeed Chuang Tsu. Did Chuang Tsu dream he was a butterfly, or did the butterfly dream he was Chuang Tsu?
>
> *(Feng and English 2008, p. 48)*

Here, we see Zhuangzi slipping between the realms of the conscious and the unconscious; between self and other. This oft-quoted dream narrative conveys an ontological and epistemological ambiguity that is so central to classical Daoist thought and proposes an inherent psychological freedom.

Personally, I believe the comparisons between Daoism and Lying Flat are ultimately superficial. The Lying Flat anti-movement is largely characterised by anxiety, exhaustion and disillusionment, whereas Daoism remains centred around the qualities of serenity, revitalisation and authenticity. One lies flat because both body and mind are alienated and exhausted, by contrast, Daoist cultivation seeks reconnection with and revitalisation of one's body, mind and spirit.

Alternative Ways of 'Dropping Out' – Dancing Away with the Seven Sages

The Daoist-inspired, Seven Sages of the Bamboo Grove are arguably China's patron saints of 'dropping out' – archetypes of freedom dancing deep within the Chinese collective unconscious. Each of the Seven Sages was formerly an important or notable figure during the politically complex and often chaotic age of the Three Kingdoms (220–280CE); a time of great division and bloodshed.

The seven sought and briefly found solace from the intrigues, dangers and hypocrisy of courtly life in the natural settings of a bamboo grove located in

Shangyang, near the home of one of the leading sages – the musician, poet and philosopher Ji Kang. There they famously engaged in wine drinking, philosophical conversation, poetic composition and recitation, and musical performances which occasionally led to shocking scenes of wild abandonment and even naked dancing. In many ways, they may be seen as constituting an early template for a countercultural ideal, one that has more than a little resonance with the famous Western countercultural movements of the 1960s. The seven sages also embodied a spirit of emboldened, unapologetic experimentation with music, spirituality and even mind-altering substances. One possible explanation for their occasional nakedness may actually relate to the use of a potent psychoactive five-mineral powder *wu shi san* 五石散, of which one of the side effects could be elevated body temperature leading to excessive sweating.

The seven came to personify the Daoist ideal of *xiao yao* 逍遙 untroubled ease, or a spirit of free and easy wandering – the term also evokes the idea, or ideal, of taking flight. They lived on as popular subjects in both Chinese and Japanese art, admired for their creativity, their independent mindedness and unwillingness to conform to societal norms and expectations – the very qualities artists often strive to embody. In the Japanese Zen monk and artist Sesson Shūkei's (1504–1589 CE) hanging scroll painting of the Seven Sages (Metropolitan Museum 2024), one encounters a merry band of carefree souls, loosely attired, ecstatically enraptured in a musical reverie, accompanied by women and children. It is significant that even the painting style and composition elements employed by Sesson were considered unorthodox at the time, further enhancing his own reputation as an eccentric. Sesson's own age, the Muromachi period in Japan, was also marked by political upheaval, in addition to artistic innovation.

In trying times of mass conformity where obedience, sycophancy and mediocrity become the prevailing norms, being eccentric becomes a revolutionary act.

The Way to *Wuwei* – Effortlessness

One of the most well-known and increasingly promoted principles of Daoism is *wu wei* 無為 commonly translated as non-action or non-doing. At first, this may seem reminiscent or evocative of the central sentiment of the 'Lying Flat' anti-movement, as it too appears to promote inaction and inactivity, but the Daoist meaning is far more nuanced and complex, as explained in Chapter 48 of the Dao De Jing, it is 'a nondoing that leaves nothing undone' (Ziporyn 2023, p. 59).

Wu wei typically encapsulates the wisdom of leaving well alone, letting be, knowing when and how to step away or back from a situation. Increasingly *wuwei* may appear as an effective alternative or antidote to our culture's promotion of perpetual busyness. Rather than an apathetic abrogation of responsibilities, *wuwei* is rooted in an understanding, often born of hard-won experience, that all too often our attempts to control or change events often only serve to further complicate and exacerbate the situation further. Our habitual tendencies to tinker our meddling mindsets can make non-action very challenging, even anxiety-inducing. In sinologist Edward Slingerland's (2014) philosophical and psychological exploration of the topic, he introduces *wu wei* with the intentionally paradoxical title 'Trying Not To Try'.

Slingerland's approach to *wu wei* is largely informed by cognitive psychology, and he often characterises the *wu wei* way of being and knowing as more intuitive, emotionally attuned and spontaneous – technically termed type i or hot cognition, in tune with the aforementioned wisdom of the gut. This is contrasted with type ii, cold cognition, which is more cerebral, processed and analytical, and is also the dominant way of thinking in and about the modern world – particularly prevalent in academia and mainstream psychological approaches.

In seeking to exemplify *wu wei*, Slingerland returns to Zhuangzi's 'Inner Chapters' and tells the tale of the virtuosic butcher Ting. The local Lord Wenhui is astounded at how the butcher can so skilfully and effortlessly cut the oxen carcass into the most desired cuts of meat. Ting's blade always moves along and through the path of least resistance, leaving his blade seemingly, miraculously untarnished and (after so many years of use) unblunted – like Ting's blade, we may also learn to move through life in a similar manner. Ting briefly recounts to his astonished Lord, the tale of how he attained his virtuosity in a short verse:

> When I first began cutting up oxen, all I could see was the ox itself. After three years, I no longer saw the ox as a whole. And now – now I meet it with my spirit and don't look with my eyes. My senses and conscious awareness have shut down and my spiritual desires take me away. I follow the Heavenly pattern of the ox, thrusting into the big hollows, guiding the knife through the big openings, and adapting my motions to the fixed structure of the ox. In this way, I never touch the smallest ligament or tendon, much less a main joint.
>
> *(Zhuangzi quoted in Slingerland 2014, p. 20)*

Significantly, we may understand this verse as illustrating a gradual movement from cold to hot cognition – transforming from a self-conscious categorising of the ox carcass accompanied by methodical movements and slices to something more akin to an ecstatic dance with or even 'flow' (Csikszentmihalyi 1989) within the Dao.

Wu wei is multifaceted and may, in the context of self-cultivation, also convey a quality of effortlessness and virtuosity – where the level of skill is so advanced that he or she makes it appear nothing much is really happening, or at the very least nothing special or extra is being added. One may think of a great artist who makes everything look so easy – who with a few seemingly simple brushstrokes can paint a living landscape. In these instances, such skill appears completely natural and utterly uncontrived, an extension or expression of one's essential nature. One does just enough and no more, and when one's task is completed, one leaves without needing nor seeking any further fanfare, thanks or adulation.

Leaving with Laozi and Taking Flight with the Immortals

By the time we encounter Laozi, the mysterious, mythic, primordial master of Daoism, the author to whom the *Dao De Jing* is traditionally attributed, he is already leaving. The most famous and familiar depictions of Laozi are of him riding away on an ox, highly reminiscent of the popular ox-herding illustrations of the Zen tradition discussed in our previous chapter. Prior to his leaving through the Hangu pass, Laozi had composed the *Dao De Jing*, upon receiving an earnest request from Yinxi, the guardian of the pass. Yinxi clearly held the former court librarian and archivist in very high esteem and felt his wisdom needed to be preserved for posterity. After this episode, Laozi appears to simply disappear without a trace, seemingly wishing to escape any mention in the very archives he had once preserved, almost as if he didn't wish to burden history with his presence.

His reasons for leaving appear to have been due to a deep sense of disillusionment with the Zhou dynasty (1046–256 BCE), which was then rapidly passing into a state of decline. Were it not for the *Dao De Jing*, it is likely that the name of Laozi would have been long forgotten, indeed this might have been his original intention. In seeking to be forgotten, he was remembered for millennia. Themes of disillusionment and forgetting pervade the Daoist teachings and hagiographies.

The common cravings for status and success are consistently mocked and subverted. In one such hagiographic tale concerning the origins of the Daoist immortal Lu Dongbin (Wong 2001), the young, mortal, aspiring scholar meets a hermit in a tavern, who unbeknownst to him is actually the Daoist immortal Zhongli Quan in disguise. The hermit invites the young man to accompany him to engage in spiritual cultivation – an invitation that he politely declines. As his meal of yellow millet is cooking, Lu Dongbin drifts into sleep and has a particularly vivid dream, what Carl Jung would have termed a 'Big Dream'. In his dream, he attains all the worldly success he had ever desired – success in the imperial exams, the highest office in the imperial court, and a beautiful wife and family. Soon however, the dream takes a dark turn, as the wheel of fate turns and his fortunes are reversed, he proceeds to lose everything he had worked so hard for and everyone he had ever loved. Upon awakening, he was amazed to learn that what he had experienced in dream time as the passage of eighteen years had in reality only been a few passing moments; the exact amount of time for his yellow millet to be cooked. Waking from his dream, Lu Dongbin simultaneously awakens from and abandons all of his worldly ambitions, resolutely determining to seek transcendence, following in the path of Zhongli Quan. Both Zhongli Quan and Lu Dongbin proceeded to become two of the famous Eight Immortals whose images adorn Daoist temples to this day.

The Eight Immortals in particular, and Daoist immortals in general, embody transcendence, with their characteristic lightness and laughter, only occasionally sighted by the righteous, riding upon the wind, clouds or cranes.

The familiar Chinese term for an immortal *xian* 仙 literally translates to 'person of the mountains'. To this day, mountains remain an integral part of the sacred geography of China and the preferred destination for hermits (both Daoist and Buddhist) to practice their spiritual cultivation.

Hermits occupy a special place in Chinese culture, as revered renunciates, seekers of deeper truths, and widely celebrated as those who are no longer blinded, bound or distracted by the red dust of worldly desires and preoccupations. The ascending of the mountains becomes synonymous with a return to nature and a recovery of authenticity. Paradoxically through seeking to abandon ambition and status, Chinese hermits have often become sought-out and revered by the emperors of all ages:

> Out of touch with the times but not with the seasons, they cultivated roots of the spirit, trading flatland dust for mountain mist. Distant and insignificant, they were the most respected men and women in the world's oldest society.
>
> *(Porter 1993, p. 1)*

The perennial fantasy of 'leaving it all behind', the allure of escape, is a universal yearning that one may easily empathise and identify with, and yet the realities of renunciation may be sobering, harsh and unforgiving, presenting many unforeseen challenges.

During the global pandemic, with its lockdowns and legally enforced quarantines, many were introduced, perhaps for the first time, to the existential challenges of stillness. Psychological Societies and Psychotherapists repeatedly warned us about the consequences of prolonged social isolation – the increased risks of resultant anxiety and depression. In one more optimistic paper, Pietrabissa and Simpson (2020) highlighted people's resilience and flexibility, paraphrasing the 78th chapter of the Dao De Jing:

> The human being – by nature – is extremely flexible – facilitating adjustment to the reality that change will become the new normality . . .
>
> In Lao Tzu's words, 'Water is fluid, soft, and yielding. But water will wear away rock, which is rigid and cannot yield. As a rule, whatever is fluid, soft and yielding will overcome whatever is rigid and hard. This is another paradox: what is soft is strong.'
>
> *(Ibid., p. 3)*

For many, however, it was a traumatising period of anxiety-inducing disconnection, feeling 'cut off' from loved ones and from one's normal, daily life. The emergent discourse of 'the new normal' belied people's struggles to adapt to these dramatic changes in their working and social lives.

When involuntary, solitude can swiftly become an unbearable burden, and life can begin to seem unliveable. It is important to remember that many hermits in the Buddhist and Daoist traditions had already engaged in intensive contemplative training prior to adopting more ascetic lifestyles in their forests, caves or mountains – in this sense the hermitage is a place of and for advanced practice, never intended for novices.

For the Daoist, stillness is actively sought and consciously cultivated as opposed to being externally imposed. Additionally, and most importantly, the Daoist adept is at ease precisely because he or she does not feel disconnected whilst in solitude but remains intimately connected. The Daoist body is not a body apart and isolated from the world and others, but is vividly reimagined and visualised as a rich, animated microcosm, containing the entire universe. In the *nei jing tu* 內經圖 inner landscape charts used by Daoist alchemists and cultivators, one can see the physiological shape of the body and its organs morph into an imaginal, geographical and astronomical realm of mountains and rivers, constellations and deities (Komjathy 2008, 2009). As the noted Daoist priest and scholar Kristopher Schipper (1993) observed, 'The human body is the image of a country' (Ibid., p. 100). It is stillness that allows one to first discover and then navigate this country.

Seeking Stillness in an Ever-Moving World

In many ways, Daoism would appear to offer an enticing alternative to the frenzied pace of modern life that so frequently frustrates and exhausts us. The slow living movement appears to share and embody many principles and practices that are foundational to a Daoist world view, particularly in regard to seeking stillness.

The quality of stillness holds a privileged position in Daoist cultivation. Stillness is the gateway to serenity, clarity, harmony and authenticity. The Chinese term for stillness, *jing* 静, can also be translated as serenity:

> Daoism has always emphasized mental serenity and maintained that good effects will come about from it. To be serene means that the mind is clear (清), or free of any thoughts that confuse it; it also means that the mind is calm (*jing* 静), without any emotions that agitate it. Daoism maintains that you should foster serenity at all times and in all activities. Activity itself is best limited to only what is most natural (*ziran* 自然) and necessary – 'nonaction' (*wuwei* 無為) is thus frequently enjoined.
>
> *(Eskildsen 2015, p. 1)*

One of the central scriptures in the popular *Quan Zhen* – Complete Reality School of Daoism, which is still commonly recited as part of the daily devotions, is titled the *Qing Jing Jing* 清静經, the 'scripture of clarity and stillness' (Komjathy 2013). This scripture enjoins and directs the adherent towards a cultivated state of serenity that leads to rediscovering and recovering an inherent harmony with the Dao.

Daoist meditation practices are arguably far less well-known than Buddhist systems, though they share many commonalities – particularly with Chinese *Chan* and Japanese *Zen*. The central element of Daoist meditation involves cultivating a state that to Western ears and sentiments might at first sound off-putting – *zuo wang* 坐忘 typically translated as 'sitting and forgetting' or the even more dramatic translation 'sitting in oblivion' (Kohn 2010).

At first, this might sound like the very opposite of mindfulness. With *Sati* Mindfulness, the etymological roots relate to memory, recollection and awareness. *Wang* 忘 as forgetfulness or oblivion may seem more counter-intuitive, less desirable or even frightening – but this state is intended to counter the greedy, binging mind, a consciousness which consumes to excess. A related name for this practice is also related to diet *xin zhai* 心齋 mind fasting.

One is not seeking to *gain* anything from the practice but to *lose* everything that is excessive. This is clarified in the 48th chapter of the Dao De Jing:

> In the pursuit of learning, every day something is acquired.
> In the pursuit of Tao, every day something is dropped.
>
> (Feng and English 1996)

The more one drops the more one may discover. What is being described is equivalent to a process of apophatic emptying (Saso 2015). Laozi reminds us that it is the emptiness of the cup that makes it useful and the hole at the wheel's centre that allows it to turn. With practice one learns to be within the 'pivot of the Dao' or the 'still-point' (Feng and English 2008, p. 29). Whereas Buddhism seeks liberation through leaving the wheel of life, the Daoist finds transcendence through placing themselves within the still-point of the turning wheel's centre.

This stillness also refers to a *transcognitive* state, before or beyond one's thoughts. In the lesser-known Daoist text *Nei Ye* 內業 (Inward Training), this is described as the 'mind within a mind', consisting of 'an awareness that precedes words' (Roth 1999, p. 117).

When one is sitting in stillness and silence, when one is no longer deafened or distracted by the 'five sounds', one can begin to more clearly discern the 'Voice of the Earth' (Roszak 1992) and tune in to the 'music of nature' (Chinn 2013, p. 25). Consequently, the artificially imposed disciplinary divisions between psychology and ecology become ever more permeable, and one's ultimate guide towards restoring harmony and authenticity becomes the natural world itself. The return to nature is itself understood to be a natural function of the Dao, as explained in the 25th chapter of the Dao De Jing:

> Humankind follows Earth,
> Earth follows Heaven,
> Heaven follows the Dao,
> The Dao follows Nature.
> (Feng and English 1996)

In the original Chinese, the word translated as nature is *zi ran* 自然, referring more broadly to inherent qualities of naturalness and spontaneity. *Zi ran* is intimately related to *wu wei*, as both are expressed through the psychological qualities of selflessness and desirelessness. These particular forms of selflessness and desirelessness may refer to a conscious process of decentring away from *ego*centric modes of having, and re-centring towards more *eco*centric modes of being.

An early ecopsychological approach is exemplified in the seventeenth-century Daoist scholar Liu Yiming's 'Awakening to the Tao' (Cleary 1988), which primarily consists of observations of the natural world which are transformed into philosophical and practical teachings:

> When turtles hide in the mud, they come to no harm. When they emerge from the mud, people catch them. When fish lurk in the depths, they remain whole. When they come out of the depths, birds kill them.
>
> What I realise as I observe this is the Tao of harming life and enhancing life.
> *(Ibid., pp. 65–66)*

The commentary proceeds to warn against conspicuously showing off one's intelligence or abilities in order to avoid being used and abused, in much the same manner Zhuangzi's oak tree recognised the wisdom of appearing useless. The key principle appears to be whether one chooses to read Zhuangzi or watch turtles at play in the mud, the same timeless lessons of the Dao are being imparted.

Learning from Turtles

A more revolutionary approach to Daoism may be encountered in Yun Rou's 'Mad Monk Manifesto' in which he resolutely critiques our 'speed and greed culture' (Yun Rou 2018, p. 100), offering an alternative model and motto – 'anything worth doing is worth doing slowly' (Ibid., p. 102).

In addition to being an ordained Daoist monk, Yun Rou has also spent over fifty years rearing and caring for turtles. While Cittaslow chose the snail as their movement's logo, the turtle is an ideal Chinese symbol for slow living. In Chinese and Daoist symbolism, the turtle represents harmony between Heaven, Earth and Humanity in addition to being an auspicious and endearing emblem of longevity. Due to their endangered status, images of turtles are increasingly frequently used by environmental movements to raise awareness concerning the urgent need for marine conservation.

Following his manifesto, Yun Rou (2020) proceeded to pen 'Turtle Planet: Compassion, Conservation and the Fate of the Natural World' in which he presents Daoism as one of the earliest expressions of an environmental consciousness.

The emulation of the turtle can also be seen in Daoist cultivation techniques such as turtle breathing (another method of embryonic breathing), where one intentionally slows and deepens one's breath to aid healing and promote longevity – but it is also the slow, deliberate, pace and placid temperament of the turtle that promotes a more wise and mindful way of being. Yun Rou explains,

> Unless we choose to live more wisely and with greater awareness, we will continue to be propelled forward without savoring the space between the notes in the music of life. Without indulging those pauses – in which lies our most profound sense of being – the melody is lost. We all know how the story ends – we get old, we get sick, we die – so what's the hurry?
>
> *(Yun Rou 2018, p. 99)*

References

Bandurski, D. (2021) The lying flat movement standing in the way of China's innovation drive. *The Brookings Institute – Tech Stream* [Online]. Available at: www.brookings.edu/techstream/the-lying-flat-movement-standing-in-the-way-of-chinas-innovation-drive/ (Accessed 21 June 2023).

Brooker, M. (2021) China isn't going to take this lying down. *Bloomberg UK* [Online]. Available at: www.bloomberg.com/opinion/articles/2021-06-19/china-s-leaders-won-t-take-a-growing-movement-of-young-slackers-lying-down (Accessed 21 June 2023).

Chinn, M. (2013) Sensing the wind: The timely music of nature's melody. *Environmental Philosophy*, 10(1), pp. 25–38.
Cleary, T. (1988) *Awakening to the Tao*. Boston, MA: Shambhala.
Cohen, E. (2011) Daoism, psychology and psychosomanautics. In: Kohn, L. (Ed.) *Living Authentically: Daoist Contributions to Modern Psychology*. Dunedin: Three Pines Press, pp. 101–122.
Csikszentmihalyi, M. (1989) *Flow: The Psychology of Optimal Experience*. New York: Harper and Row.
Eskildsen, S. (2015) *Daoism, Meditation and the Wonders of Serenity*. New York: State University of New York Press.
Feng, G. and English, J. (1996) *Tao Te Ching*. Aldershot: Gower Publishing.
Feng, G. and English, J. (2008) *Chuang Tsu Inner Chapters: A Companion Volume to Tao Te Ching*. Portland: Amber Lotus Publishing.
Gershon, M. D. (2019) *The Second Brain: The Scientific Basis of Gut Instinct and a Groundbreaking New Understanding of Nervous Disorders of the Stomach and Intestine*. New York: HarperCollins.
Graham, A. C. (1990) *The Book of Lieh-tzŭ: A Classic of the Tao*. New York: Columbia University Press.
Kohn, L. (2010) *Daoist Dietetics: Food for Immortality*. Honolulu, HI: University of Hawaii Press.
Kohn, L. (2011) *Living Authentically: Daoist Contributions to Modern Psychology*. Dunedin, FL: Three Pines Press.
Komjathy, L. (2008) Mapping the daoist body (1): The *Neijing tu* in history. *Journal of Daoist Studies*, 1, pp. 67–92.
Komjathy, L. (2009) Mapping the daoist body (2): The text of the *Neijing tu*. *Journal of Daoist Studies*, 2, pp. 64–108.
Komjathy, L. (2013) *The Way of Complete Perfection: A Quanzhen Daoist Anthology*. New York: SUNY Press.
Koon, W. K. (2021) Why are young Chinese people being criticised for lying flat? It proved an invaluable cultural gain for the country once. *South China Morning Post* [Online]. Available at: www.scmp.com/magazines/post-magazine/article/3138431/why-are-young-chinese-people-criticised-lying-flat-it (Accessed 21 June 2023).
Maciocia, G. (2015) *The Foundations of Chinese Medicine: A Comprehensive Text* (3rd ed.). New York: Elsevier.
Maslow, A. (1993) *The Farther Reaches of Human Nature*. New York: Penguin Arkana.
Metropolitan Museum (2024) Seven sages of the bamboo grove [Online]. Available at: www.metmuseum.org/art/collection/search/53231 (Accessed 20 February 2023).
Peng, K., Spencer-Rodgers, J. and Nian, Z. (2006) Naïve dialecticism and the Tao of Chinese thought. In: Kim, U., Yang, K. and Hwang, K. (Eds.) *Indigenous and Cultural Psychology: Understanding People in Context*, New York: Springer. pp. 247–262.
Pietrabissa, G. and Simpson, S. (2020) Psychological consequences of social isolation during COVID-19 outbreak. *Frontiers in Psychology*, 11, Article 2201.
Porter, B. (1993) *Road to Heaven: Encounters with Chinese Hermits*. San Francisco, CA: Mercury House.
Roszak, T. (1992) *The Voice of the Earth: An Exploration of Ecopsychology*. New York: Simon & Schuster.
Roth, H. (1999) *Original Tao: Inward Training (Nei-yeh) and the Foundations of Taoist Mysticism*. New York: Columbia University Press.
Saso, M. (2012) *The Teachings of Daoist Master Zhuang*. Los Angeles, CA: Oracle Bone Press.
Saso, M. (2015) *Mystic, Shaman, Oracle, Priest: Prayer without Words*. Pacific Grove, CA: Sino-Asian Institute of America.
Schipper, K. (1993) *The Taoist Body*. Berkeley, CA: University of California Press.

Slingerland, E. (2014) *Trying Not to Try: The Art of Effortlessness and the Power of Spontaneity*. Edinburgh: Canongate Books.
Slosar, J. R. (2009) *The Culture of Excess: How America Lost Self-Control and Why We Need to Redefine Success*. Westport, CT: Greenwood Publishing.
Wang, M. (2011) *Foundations of Inner Alchemy: The Taoist Practice of Neidan* (Trans. Pregadio, F.). Mountain View, CA: Golden Elixir Press.
Ward, J. E. (2007) *Chinese Memories*. Morrisville, NC: Lulu Publishing.
Welwood, J. (1979) *The Meeting of the Ways: Explorations in East/West Psychology*. New York: Shocken Books.
Wong, E. (2001) *Tales of the Taoist Immortals*. Boulder, CO: Shambhala Publications.
Yun Rou (2018) *Mad Monk Manifesto: A Prescription for Evolution, Revolution and Global Awakening*. Coral Gables, FL: Mango Publishing Group.
Yun Rou (2020) *Turtle Planet: Compassion, Conservation and the Fate of the Natural World*. Coral Gables, FL: Mango Publishing.
Zhang, Z. and Li, K. (2023) So you choose to "Lie Flat?" "Sang-ness," affective economies, and the "Lying Flat" movement. *Quarterly Journal of Speech*, 109(1), pp. 48–69.
Ziporyn, B. (2023) *Daodejing: Laozi*. New York: Liveright Publishing.

5

REDISCOVERING AND RECLAIMING THE PACE OF NATURE

Cohen and Eichenbaum (1994) astutely observed that 'as soon as one turns to biology, it becomes apparent that wheels do not exist anywhere in nature' (Ibid., p. 6).

Despite this, the world, effortlessly and imperceptibly, continues to turn.

Long before the invention of the wheel, the circular and cyclical pervaded and shaped our sense of time and space. Seasons and phases, waxings and wanings, dawns and dusks, each stemming from and seamlessly blending into one another – just as our lives are maintained by the continuous rhythm of the rising and falling of our breath.

Today, we find ourselves inextricably bound to the wheel of 'clock time'. Our lives are artificially measured and governed by ticks and chimes, electronic alerts, reminders and alarms. We race and strive to save time, we commodify time, parroting questionable aphorisms such as 'time is money'. Whether it is the latest sale, our tax returns, or the impending climate crisis, we seem to be being constantly reminded of scarcity that 'time is running out'. We may consequently find ourselves becoming deadened and desensitised to a life of looming deadlines. Such a blinkered, temporal bondage makes us so much less than we truly are – it is worth remembering that the word 'minute' may, depending on its context, refer to both a short unit of time and a small scale of size.

The French philosopher Henri Bergson understood that our failure to meaningly reflect on time could lead to an impoverished, partially lived life. Bergson distinguished between two types of time – *temps*, referring to our constructed (and constrictive), consensus consciousness of clock-time, and

DOI: 10.4324/9781003334972-5

the *durée*, referring to a more natural, organic flow of time which cannot be measured but can only be experientially encountered and lived.

> According to Bergson, human time might be reclaimed from the physicists by philosophers and poets convinced that life is growth through metamorphosis rather than 'construction', contraries rather than concatenation.
> *(Douglass 1986, p. 12)*

In Bergson's dialogues with Albert Einstein, he uses the language and experience of listening to music to better understand time – 'Melody, now, is also the metaphor par excellence by which Bergson elucidates his concept of duration. Duration is the cornerstone of Bergson's philosophy' (Posman 2012, p. 108). If we persist in measuring and living our lives according to the artificial, monotonous metronome of *temps*, we risk missing the timeless, meditative melody of *durée*.

If, however, we can begin to gradually extricate ourselves from our habitual tendencies to view time through a purely quantitative frame, then we might catch transformative glimpses of new heightened realities, famously described by Blake in his 'Auguries of Innocence':

> To see a world in a grain of sand
> And a heaven in a wild flower
> Hold infinity in the palm of your hand
> And eternity in an hour.
> A Robin Red breast in a cage
> Puts all heaven in a rage.
> (Blake 1982, p. 490)

As one of the foremost romantic poets, Blake passionately advocated for a return to nature and innocence in order to recover and rediscover ourselves – it is in nature that we find ourselves freed from our collective cages. One may justifiably question whether any authentic 'return to innocence' is still possible in this increasingly synthetic and digital age.

The poem's title 'Auguries' refers to ancient Roman divinatory practices of observing the flight patterns and behaviour of birds, and one might consider how human activity continues to detrimentally affect and deplete their habitats, disrupting their natural cycles and threatening their very survival (French and Rockwell 2011).

My very first academic paper explored some of the overlaps between Daoism and Environmental Psychology, and in it I had also included a particularly troubling example of changing avian behaviour:

> When Britain voted for its favourite wildlife clip from Sir David Attenborough's long and illustrious career (Natural History Museum Poll,

> April 15th, 2006), it chose footage of the South Australian Lyrebird which somehow manages to distinguish between and perfectly imitate all the animal calls it hears in its habitat (the rainforests of New South Wales).
>
> In the past the bird had been recorded flawlessly mimicking the mating calls and sounds of other birds and animals (Reilly 1988). However, recently, a more disturbing behaviour had been recorded. It seemed the bird was now imitating the sounds of camera shutters, mobile phones, car alarms and even chainsaws (the very chainsaws that were destroying its habitat).
>
> Footage of the Lyrebird imitating the chainsaw was shown during one of Sir David Attenborough's interviews with Michael Parkinson (BBC1, June 16th, 2007) and seemed to stir Attenborough to his core. In his famously familiar and hushed tones he suggested that the bird unknowingly 'sings the song of its own demise'.
>
> *(Cohen 2008, pp. 36–37)*

In our previous chapter, we considered how the Daoist seeks to tune into the music of nature, but now we need to consider how we, as a species, are actively and irrevocably transforming the Earth's soundscapes – unconsciously composing the symphony of our own destruction.

Our current age is commonly referred to as the 'Anthropocene' by climate scientists, geologists, ecologists and archaeologists. It describes the dawning of new geological era, beginning around the same time as the first industrial revolution. To refer to the Anthropocene implies an acceptance that human activity is now having a direct, detrimental and measurable impact on our planet's climate and ecosystems. This impact includes transforming the very sound of our planet. One recent headline in the *Wall Street Journal* noted that 'Astronomers Can't Hear Signals From Space Because Earth Is Too Loud' (Winning 2021) and proceeded 'Radio pulses from exploded stars are no match for cellphone towers, faulty toilets and microwave ovens shouting in your ear' (Ibid.)

In Bernie Krause's (2012) thought-provoking study of the natural origins of music, he explores the sounds, songs and rhythms of the Earth and all living beings – he terms these naturally arising sounds Geophony and Biophony – etymologically evoking 'the voice of the Earth' and 'voice of life'. Over forty years of recording wild soundscapes and over fifteen thousand species, Krause regrets that due to human activity over half the sounds he recorded for his archive are now no longer audible in our world. Our own cacophonous contribution to 'The Great Animal Orchestra' (Ibid. 2012), the anthropophony of the Anthropocene, appears to have drowned out and forever silenced a great many voices.

In addition to the deafening effects of the anthropophony, we are being increasingly blinded by our own light pollution. As well as being the bane of astronomers worldwide, struggling to locate stars and planetary bodies above the sickly orange glow of streetlights, the excess light that human beings produce is having diverse and detrimental effects, ranging from disturbing our sleep cycles to disrupting turtle and bird migration and mating patterns. In a related documentary 'The City Dark' (Cheney 2011), scientists reflect on the psychological consequences of losing the night sky, which includes losing our sense of scale, perspective and place in the universe. The great cosmologist Carl Sagan famously referred to Earth as 'The Pale Blue Dot' (Sagan 2011) and emphasised our need for increased humility and humanity when faced with the unimaginable vastness, antiquity and indifference of the cosmos. Failure or the inability to even see, let alone face and contemplate the cosmos and our place in it, may only serve to further amplify our anthropocentric and egocentric world views – continuing to place our species and ourselves at the centre of *our* known universe. However, Sagan's and many contemporary scientists' presentation of a cold, indifferent universe carries its own risks. We might use this stark vision to further justify and rationalise our own anthropocentric apathy as being a natural inheritance, reflection or consequence of a greater cosmic indifference. As Sagan so memorably mused in his groundbreaking series Cosmos:

> The cosmos is also within us. We're made of star-stuff. We are a way for the cosmos to know itself.
>
> *(Sagan 1980)*

Thus, we might mitigate this risk by remembering that if we are indeed a living part of our universe then the universe is only truly as indifferent as we allow ourselves to become. When it comes to the natural world, one does not simply encounter apathy and indifference, one often encounters great passion, a profound sense of wonder, connection and appreciation, and of course love.

Biophilia

The term biophilia is first found in Erich Fromm's (1973) 'Anatomy of Human Destructiveness', where he described it as a passionate love of all that lives. The term was further developed and re-presented as the 'biophilia hypothesis' by Kellert and Wilson (1993). The biophilia hypothesis proposes that human beings possess an instinctual drive to seek connection and affiliation with the natural world. An even earlier, more poetic expression of biophilia can be found in the writings of the much-revered American Transcendentalist Ralph Waldo Emerson. In his 1884 essay 'Nature', Emerson emotes:

> We never can part with it; the mind loves its old home: as water to our thirst, so is the rock, the ground, to our eyes, and hands, and feet. It is firm water: it is cold flame: what health, what affinity!
>
> *(Emerson 1995, p. 261)*

For the American Transcendentalists and the English Romantics, nature is not merely our love, but occupies a more hallowed position as our first, original love.

The nature of this love is also worth considering further, particularly in regard to the Ancient Greek term *philia* φιλία. Unfortunately, the suffixes *phile* and *philia* have become somewhat soiled in recent times and are commonly associated with unnatural, excessive or pathological forms of desire. It is important to remember that *philia* traditionally referred to love and friendship.

In the Nicomachean Ethics (340 BCE), Aristotle outlined different types of friendship. Friendship necessarily begins within oneself – that is to say, loving another as one loves oneself, and seeing one's self reflected in another. This may lead to a more altruistic love, which Aristotle compares to the love a mother has for her son. In Rhetoric II 4, Aristotle proceeds to describe *philia* as 'wanting for someone what one thinks good, for his sake and not for one's own, and being inclined, so far as one can, to do such things for him' (Aristotle quoted in Gartner 2017, p. 147).

But to what extent do we *still* see ourselves reflected in the natural world, or harbour any such selfless sentiments towards Mother Nature?

When one considers the current climate emergency resulting from the destructive and exploitative relationship we have with our natural world, it becomes ever more difficult to relate to biophilia in this more ancient and altruistic sense of the word. In a manner not too dissimilar from the way the suffixes *philia* and *phile* became increasingly pathologised, divorced from friendship and love, so too has our relationship with the natural world arguably deteriorated from nurturing to abusive. Ecofeminists have even referred to the act of sexual assault to characterise this destructive dynamic, protesting the rape of the Earth (Sturgeon 1997).

When James Lovelock (1979) first proposed his paradigm-shifting Gaia Hypothesis, he argued that we must begin to see and perceive the world as an immense and ancient, living, breathing organism, with the hope that this might fundamentally change our attitudes towards and relationship with our planet. Towards this end, we may necessarily need to recover some of the pre-modern, animistic veneration towards nature that our ancestors naturally possessed and that many indigenous peoples still express – both the love and the awe.

In Ancient Greek mythology, Gaia is the very first, primordial Goddess to emerge from Chaos – older than all the Titans of Mount Othrys and the later Gods of Mount Olympus. Modern representations of Gaia as Mother Earth tend to follow the rather romanticised convention of focusing almost exclusively on her beauty, bountiful and nurturing nature, but in doing so miss, reduce or repress her more ambivalent nature.

In the living traditions of Goddess worship in India, the Divine Feminine is understood as being both the creator and the destroyer. The gentle, benignly smiling protector Mahadevi (the supreme Goddess) is one and the same as the

Goddess Kali, who dances wildly and mercilessly upon the crushed corpses of demonic forces. Those who would adore and venerate the Goddess in her benevolent form must also recollect and respect her wrathful form – the wild, fanged ferocity of a loving mother protecting her children.

The term Biophilia entered a more popular, public consciousness with the global release of the Icelandic musician Björk's (2011) innovative and interactive app-album 'Biophilia', which included guest narrations from the nation's favourite naturalist, David Attenborough. Together, they sought to creatively explore and raise awareness of the relationships between nature, music and technology. In addition to her embrace of electronic (electronica) and technological (techno) sound, Björk's music has also often sought to incorporate the geophonies of her native Iceland – from explosive volcanic beats to ethereal, glacial chimes and stirring string arrangements, providing an artistic template for a more harmonious relationship between technology and ecology.

In introducing his recent Netflix nature documentary series 'Our Planet', David Attenborough delivered a speech at the event premiere, which included the following unsettling observation:

> Nature once determined how we survive. Now we determine how nature survives. One of the things Darwin's work has taught us, is that we break nature's connections at our peril. Yet break them we do – at ever greater speed.
>
> *(Attenborough 2019)*

Perhaps the heart of the problem lies in the all too casual, unacknowledged, possessive language of *our* planet.

We habitually visualise ourselves at and as the centre of our world, or in the case of Aristotle's influential *scala naturae* – ladder of nature, standing above and looking down upon the animals and plants of the natural world. But Nature is neither a wheel nor a ladder, we are neither at its centre nor bestriding its top. For some time, ecologists have preferred to represent ecosystems as a living, expansive *web* of life, consisting of a great many complex interconnected threads.

Ecologists are keen to stress our interconnectivity, for Deep Ecologists, this relationship takes on a deeper, more spiritual character, emphasising interdependence. Arne Naess, one of the founding figures of Deep Ecology, proposed an enlarged, interconnected, cosmic sense of self, inspired by the Hindu concept of Atman:

> Through the wider self every living being is connected intimately and from this intimacy follows the capacity of identification, and as its natural consequence, the practice of non-violence.
>
> *(Naess 1987, p. 25)*

Esteemed environmental activist Gary Snyder, widely acknowledged as the poet laureate of deep ecology, consistently emphasises the importance of interdependence, mainly drawing on his lifelong immersion in Buddhist traditions.

One of his most celebrated and memorable poems is the 'Smokey the Bear Sutra' (1969). Smokey the Bear remains an iconic American symbol of care for and conservation of the national forests – a popular personification of a safety campaign originally launched in 1944. His tall Teddy Bear visage is lodged deep within the American psyche – an anthropomorphised bear, carrying a shovel and wearing a park ranger's hat, points out of a poster imploring 'Remember . . . only YOU can prevent forest fires'.

Snyder's poem evokes traditional Tibetan Buddhist iconography, reimagining 'Smokey' as a wrathful protector of the Earth. The poem's introduction expresses a more biophilic sense of belonging – a belonging *with* as opposed to a belonging *to*. This leads to an *our* that pertains not to possession but to relation, transitioning from the mode of having to ways of being and inter-being – emerging from a reawakened ecological consciousness that constitutes a potent remedy for both anthropocentrism and resourcism:

> The twisting strata of the great mountains and the pulsings of volcanoes are my love burning deep in the earth. My obstinate compassion is schist and basalt and granite, to be mountains, to bring down the rain. In that future American Era I shall enter a new form; to cure the world of loveless knowledge that seeks with blind hunger: and mindless rage eating food that will not fill it.
>
> *(Snyder 1969)*

In Snyder's poem, the more local threat of forest fire becomes the global, apocalyptic 'fires of the Kali Yuga':

> fires caused by the stupidity of those who think things can be gained and lost whereas in truth all is contained vast and free in the Blue Sky and Green Earth of One Mind.
>
> *(Ibid.)*

The Sutra-like quality might bring to mind a similarly themed, earlier teaching of Buddha, known as the *Ādittapariyāya Sutta* the Fire Sermon. In this well-known sutra, the Buddha declares that the whole world is aflame with craving, burning with hatred, smoking with ignorance. Much like Smokey the Bear, the Buddha also recognises that we are primarily responsible for both our state of suffering and our own liberation – 'only YOU can prevent forest fires'. This statement is not intended to further stoke the fires of our own sense of self-importance – though we are not the centre of the world, we remain responsible for the state of our world and the state of our minds.

Seeking to challenge the 'Human Exceptionalist Paradigm', Catton and Dunlap (1978) proposed the New Environmental Paradigm (NEP) scale. A core component of the NEP recognised and emphasised humanity's place within a wider ecosystem. This recognition of humanity's alienation from the natural world continues to be discussed in more contemporary debates concerning 'Nature Deficit Disorder' (Louv 2005).

When one first hears the term 'Nature Deficit Disorder' (NDD), one might be forgiven for wanting to consult the current fifth, revised edition of the *Diagnostic and Statistical Manual of Mental Disorders* (DSM-V-TR) to search for the official listing, descriptions and symptoms of this particular disorder. Perhaps one might expect to find it being discussed alongside the far more familiar, similar sounding, sibling condition attention deficit disorder (ADD). However, there is currently no such condition as NDD to be found within the DSM. Louv's choice of clinical sounding terminology intentionally, rhetorically raises the question of whether our lack of contact with the natural world should be taken far more seriously than it currently is:

> Nature-deficit disorder describes the human costs of alienation from nature, among them: diminished use of the senses, attention difficulties, and higher rates of physical and emotional illness.
>
> *(Louv 2005, p. 36)*

In addition to this named 'nature deficit', Louv encourages us to reflect on the synthetic excess and surplus of our increasingly technocentric, technophilic lifestyles, and how, for many children, screen time indoors has replaced traditional outdoor playtime.

Louv's book is poignantly titled 'Last Child in the Woods' conveying a tragic sense of loss. It evokes collectively fading, nostalgic memories of childhood's natural rites of passage – climbing tall trees or learning how to thread daisy chains. It suggests that the child who plays outdoors, in nature, is now akin to an endangered animal, like the last remaining 'endlings' of a species on the brink of extinction.

But sentimentality alone is insufficient to make a convincing case for nature's preservation. Louv is keen to clearly illustrate the developmental, psychological and spiritual consequences resulting from our increasing disengagement with and detachment from the natural world – one endures a stunted growth and risks a significant decline in both one's physical and mental health. There are also more global, ecological consequences of NDD, beyond the personal and psychological spheres.

A central question raised by Louv's work, with far-reaching environmental implications, is 'How can we be ever expected to genuinely care *for* the natural world if we don't first cultivate any authentic sense of connection *towards* it?' This alienation from the natural world doesn't simply lead to diminishing rates of biophilia but risks a rise in biophobia – seeing and perceiving nature as something other, alien and threatening.

When Theodore Roszak (1992) outlined his 'Eight Principles of Ecopsychology', he was even more emphatic in regard to the profound psychological and environmental consequences of our continued alienation from the natural world:

> The core of the mind is the ecological unconscious. For ecopsychology, repression of the ecological unconscious is the deepest root of collusive madness in industrial society. Open access to the ecological unconscious is the path to sanity.
>
> *(Ibid., p. 320)*

Roszak continues to argue that this path to ecological consciousness is at its most accessible during childhood, as expressed in the fourth point:

> For ecopsychology as for other therapies, the crucial stage of development is the life of the child. The ecological unconscious is regenerated, as if it were a gift, in the newborn's enchanted sense of the world. Ecopsychology seeks to recover the child's innately animistic quality of experience in functionally 'sane' adults.
>
> *(Ibid.)*

From the perspectives of deep ecology and ecopsychology, our estrangement from the natural world mirrors our estrangement from ourselves and one another. Returning to the natural world offers the hopes of reconnection and restoration.

In addition to the more intuitive sense we possess concerning nature's healing properties, there is now quite a strong, established evidence base to support the numerous health benefits, both physical and psychological, of being in or near natural environments.

Pioneering studies by Roger Ulrich bolstered the biophilia hypothesis by convincingly demonstrating the stress-reducing and healing effects of the natural world – how we are both emotionally and physiologically soothed by natural features – forests, mountains and lakes. Ulrich's (1984) best-known study concerning a 'view from a window' observed how exposure to natural scenery contributed towards patients' recovery in hospitals – reducing the need for pain medication, supporting healing and reducing the duration of their stay. The 2023 winning garden of the RHS Chelsea Flower Show, 'Horatio's Garden', was designed with precisely such research in mind, to serve as an 'immersive and restorative haven' (RHS 2023) that could be viewed from a patient's bed.

Stephen and Rachel Kaplan (1989) further demonstrated how we think and feel differently in natural environments, through contrasting the ways we habitually attend to stimuli in the built environment. The apparent convenience of our daily urban lives comes with quite a heavy cognitive cost, as we are constantly required to employ focused, direct attention to the various, competing stimuli that surround us, constantly demanding our attention – from congested traffic, to hurried pedestrians, to perpetually glowing computer and phone screens. Maintaining the required level of focus to effectively function invariably/inevitably leads to fatigue, which we might further culturally contextualise through linking to 'urban exhaustion' (Madden 2022):

> Urban exhaustion results from the febrile rhythm and hastening speed of today's crisis-prone, globalised, financialised capitalism.
>
> *(Ibid.)*

Madden's description of the dehumanising pace and alienating effects of modern urban living might justifiably make one yearn for a more natural alternative. One possible, although admittedly partial answer to urban exhaustion is natural restoration, as proposed in the Kaplans' (1989) Attention Restoration Theory (ART).

As our environment transforms from looming skyscrapers and cityscapes to wide open skies, from noisy traffic to whispering trees, a potent psychological transformation may begin to take place. In a more natural setting, we downshift from a demanding, hard focus and direct attending to an effortless, more diffused 'soft fascination' (Ibid., p. 192) where the eye wanders and the mind wonders with comparative ease. As liberating as this might at first sound, in reality it is only offering a relatively brief respite before we return to the urban jungle. However restorative the natural environment may be, we eventually go home to our built environments. But what if we could bring nature back with us, by integrating more natural features into our built environments?

Biophilic Design and Salvation

Biophilic design rests on the understanding that our built environments often serve to reinforce and exacerbate our sense of alienation from the natural world, from one another and from ourselves.

There appears a general, widespread sense of dissatisfaction with the current state of urban planning and architecture. Despite the celebrated efficiency, staggering speed of construction and cost-effectiveness of modern modular design, mass-produced, prefabricated structures, they can all too often appear too sterile, homogenous and denatured – frequently emphasising and elevating utilitarian function over aesthetic form. These impersonal, dehumanised and dehumanising structures can commonly seem divorced from the natural world – they appear not only dead but deadening. In Kunze et al.'s (2014) 'Architecture Post Mortem', they propose that the current state of architecture reflects the dysphoric states of mind, distorted by late/end-stage capitalism.

A much more optimistic alternative may be encountered through the proponents of biophilic design, who summarise its central principle through the admirable aspiration of 'bringing buildings to life' (Kellert et al. 2008), in the hopes of achieving an architectural renaissance that will reinspire residents. Biophilic design looks to the natural world for its inspiration.

One of the earliest advocates and innovators of biophilic design was the Austrian-born artist Friedensreich Hundertwasser (1928–2000).

The natural world was Hundertwasser's lifelong instructor – he was even known to hold his paintings up against surrounding trees to ensure that they complemented and were congruent with the natural world. In a similar spirit to Roszak, Hundertwasser understood our separation from the natural world as constituting a primary source of collective sickness, whilst also representing a dire existential threat. For Hundertwasser, the artist's enemies were artificiality, regimentation and mass production, all products of a restrictive rationalism that he would repeatedly equate with the straight line of architectural orthodoxy.

In Hundertwasser's (1964) 'Mouldiness Manifesto Against Rationalism in Architecture', he passionately protests the proliferation and sterility of cubelike dwellings that imprison, psychologically and spiritually impoverish their inhabitants, seemingly anticipating contemporary 'prefab' trends in construction.

Hundertwasser observed how the natural world was being consistently misplaced, pushed to the periphery of our daily lives, all but excluded from the built environment. He earnestly, continuously sought to bring back and integrate the living, natural world into our homes.

A popular motto of Hundertwasser, often appearing all in capitals was that

> THE HORIZONTAL BELONGS TO NATURE, THE VERTICAL TO MAN
>
> *(Hundertwasser 1971)*

This core principle was realised through his architecture, that brought to life otherwise bare balconies, with abundant, blossoming flowers and transformed characterless grey rooftops into lush green gardens, as can still be seen in Vienna's iconic *Hundertwasserhaus*. Despite the apparent duality expressed in this motto, Hundertwasser envisioned the natural world as being an integral part of humanity's heritage and future – that human nature is very much a part of nature, as near and necessary to us as our own skin. In one of his later, smaller illustrations 'Men's Five Skins', Hundertwasser and his close friend, the French art critic and cultural philosopher Piere Restany, developed what might be interpreted as an inverted version of the traditional Daoist inner landscapes. This simple, almost childlike sketch depicts the skins of the self extending ever further outwards into the universe, seemingly illustrating Naess' 'wider self'. The first skin is our own epidermis, followed by our clothing, our second skin. Our third skin consists of our physical homes. The fourth skin refers to our social and cultural identity. The fifth and final:

> is the planetary skin, directly concerned with the fate of the biosphere, the quality of the air we breathe, and the state of the earth's crust that shelters and feeds us.
>
> *(Restany 1998, pp. 10–11)*

In a simple but visceral sense, Hundertwasser encourages us not only to see and place ourselves within the natural world but also to see nature as an intimate extension of ourselves – in this sense, biophilic design becomes a natural expression of biophilia, and biophilia becomes the primary means towards ecological salvation and spiritual redemption:

> The relationship between man and trees must gain a religious dimension and replace the adoration of Christ or God. Only when a divine adoration of all vegetation takes hold, a gradual improvement of the environment can begin from the inside of people. Then, there will also be a better understanding of the phrase: THE STRAIGHT LINE IS GODLESS.
>
> *(Hundertwasser 1971)*

The influential architect and urbanist, Christopher Alexander, had also spent a lifetime striving to naturalise, humanise and even spiritualise our built environments. He is perhaps most celebrated for his early work 'A Pattern Language' (Alexander et al. 1977), which sought to demonstrate the underlying patterns and qualities that can effectively transform sterile spaces into welcoming places.

His final, and arguably most ambitious work, 'The Nature of Order: An Essay on Architecture and The Nature of the Universe', was a four-volume opus – defining and exploring what he terms living structure and living centres (Alexander 2004). This work takes on a far more personal tone than his previous publications, and he repeatedly recognises that the reader may struggle with its more overtly spiritual content and message:

> To make the reader share with me my sense of what is really happening in the architectural examples where life appears, I shall now try to describe

> something – a feeling so remote from our ordinary sense of things, that it may have to be called *meta*-physical – truly beyond physics.
>
> *(Ibid., p. 146)*

The concluding fourth volume, 'The Luminous Ground', presents what could be fairly described as a Transpersonal approach to architecture, extending quite far beyond formal structure and into more metaphysical realms of meaning and experience. Throughout the book, Alexander repeatedly critiques the cul-de-sac of materialist and mechanistic approaches to architecture.

For Alexander, the natural world and natural forms profoundly affect us partly because we see ourselves reflected within them – a familiar sense of biophilia, but more than simply being biophilic resonance or remembrance, the natural world calls out to an 'I' that has timeless and transcendent properties:

> The rock, the ripple in the pond, and the fish darting along the stream are connected to this I, reverberate with I, awaken and enliven us, continually refresh the I that sleeps within us.
>
> *(Alexander 2004, p. 4)*

This 'I that sleeps within us' seeks connection with something timeless that exists 'in me, and before me, and after me' (Ibid., p. 5), and transpersonal, reaching out to 'the heart beyond the heart' (Ibid., p. 7) or 'eternal self' (Ibid., p. 70) – similar in scope to the Daoist's 'mind within the mind' described in Chapter 4.

The restorative and transformative potency of an architecture bourn from Alexander's vision for a new cosmology of living structure is described in a quasi-mystical manner which reaches deep beneath our skin and bestows an ecstatic, beatific state of belonging:

> It is tied to us, as if by blood. It is ours. We shine in its presence. Such a building endows us with knowledge of ourselves, makes us feel awake, conscious, more human, more ourselves, and in the end makes us experience ourselves as if dissolved in a flood of tears.
>
> *(Ibid., p. 70)*

On the page directly opposite, these words is a black and white photograph of a child (the author in his youth) – eyes closed, arm outstretched, seemingly blissfully immersed in nature, reminiscent of Louv's eponymous 'Last Child in the Woods'. Beneath the image is a caption that concisely encapsulates Roszak's earlier descriptions of the ecological unconscious – 'It is the core of the earth and child in me' (Alexander 2004, p. 71).

This deep, inner yearning to return to the natural world, to be reunited with our first love and to recover the child's sense of wonder seems more fittingly the domain of poetry than psychology or ecology, and it is through poetry and literature that we may uncover the modern roots of biophilic longing.

Returning to Our Roots – Tuning-in to the Voice of Nature

> I went to the woods because I wished to live deliberately, to front only the essential facts of life, and I see if I could not learn what it had to teach, and not, when I came to die, discover that I had not lived.
>
> (Thoreau 2004, p. 182)

These famous words from Thoreau's 'Walden' became and remain a rallying cry for Deep Ecologists, Ecopsychologists, Wilderness Therapists and Forest School educators.

Today, this quote occupies a prominent place, on a wooden sign at Walden Pond, in Concord, Massachusetts, next to the original site of the cabin, where Thoreau lived for two years, two months and two days. The duration of his retreat is reminiscent of the traditional three-year, three-month and three-day retreats undertaken by Tibetan Buddhist practitioners, seeking to deepen their commitment to the Dharma and purify their mindstreams in preparation for receiving the higher teachings. Certainly, for Thoreau, this was also a very personal pilgrimage, a spiritual quest to recover something timeless and authentic – 'To anticipate, not the sunrise and the dawn merely, but if possible, Nature herself!' (Ibid., p. 124).

His immersion in nature allows him to tune-in to the geophony of the wind, which takes on a divine or theophonic quality, conveyed through reverent prose:

> The winds which passed over my dwelling were such as sweep over the ridges of mountains, bearing the broken strains, or celestial parts only, of terrestrial music. The morning wind forever blows, the poem of creation is uninterrupted; but few are the ears that hear it. Olympus is but the outside of the earth every where.
>
> *(Ibid., p. 177)*

Thoreau's writings still retain relevance, voicing our desire to escape the rat race, travel off the beaten track, and return to nature and simplicity. One discerns a deep disillusionment with both the dehumanising effects of industrialisation and the rapidly rising tides of urbanisation.

> But lo! men have become the tools of their tools. The man who independently plucked the fruits when he was hungry is become a farmer; and he

> who stood under a tree for shelter, a housekeeper. We now no longer camp as for a night, but have settled down on earth and forgotten heaven.
>
> *(Thoreau quoted in Rosenblum 2000, p. 48)*

It is important to remember that Thoreau was living through the transportation and market revolutions of the 1820s and 1830s which were having a seismic impact upon the social, political and spiritual landscape of America. It was not merely the scale of change that concerned Thoreau, but also the pace of change:

> It lives too fast. Men think that is essential that the *Nation* have commerce, and export ice, and talk through a telegraph, and ride thirty miles an hour, without a doubt, whether *they* do or not; but whether we should live like baboons or men, is a little uncertain.
>
> *(Thoreau 2004 p. 183)*

He continues to question the point of perpetual busyness, viewing it as a form of illness:

> Why should we live with such hurry and waste of life? We are determined to be starved before we are hungry. Men say that a stitch in time saves nine, and so they take a thousand stitched to-day and save nine to-morrow. As for *work*, we haven't any of any consequence. We have the Saint Vitus' dance, and cannot possibly keep our heads still.
>
> *(Ibid.)*

This abiding aversion to speed was shared by Thoreau's friend and mentor, Ralph Waldo Emerson. Walden Pond was actually located on Emerson's estate and so one might reasonably say that both men, for a time, shared a physical as well as an intellectual landscape. Both men are celebrated as founding figures of the American Transcendentalist movement which sanctified the natural world and strived for a sacred simplicity in which humankind might rediscover their authenticity and individuality.

Emerson's spiritual sustenance owed as much to Hindu thought, as it did to the popular reforming, universalist influence of the American Unitarian Church, in which Emerson was a pastor. In 1845, the same year that Thoreau moved into his cabin at Walden Pond, Emerson was reading Charles Wilkens' first English translation of the *Bhagavad Gita*, but Vedic principles were already being expressed in his earlier essay 'The Over-Soul' (first published in 1841). Here, Emerson sought to recover the eternal, spiritual core that lies concealed within the heart of humanity – hearkening back to *Mundaka Upanishad* discussed in Chapter 2. The primary cause of this concealment appears to be an increasingly materialist outlook, and Emerson introduces the Over-Soul by way of contrast, after critiquing the prevailing physicalist world view:

> We live in succession, in division, in parts, in particles. Meantime, within man is the soul of the whole; the wise silence; the universal beauty, to which every part and particle is equally related; the eternal ONE.
>
> *(Emerson 1995, p. 131)*

Emerson shared Thoreau's belief that it is only within the natural world that we may regain our sense of the sacred. In Emerson's essay 'Nature' which was published a year before Thoreau's arrival at Walden Pond, he declares:

> Man is fallen; nature is erect, and serves as a differential thermometer, detecting the presence or absence of the divine sentiment within man.
>
> *(Emerson 1995, p. 265)*

Towards the end of the essay, Emerson expresses a comedic contempt for the acceleration of American society, which uncannily appears to predict and critique a decidedly modern-sounding fast food mentality:

> We anticipate a new era from the invention of a locomotive, or a balloon; the new engine brings with it the old checks. They say that by electro-magnetism, your salad shall be grown from the seed, whilst your fowl is roasting for dinner: it is a symbol of our modern aims and endeavours, – of our condensation and acceleration of objects: but nothing is gained: nature cannot be cheated: man's life is but seventy salads long, grow they swift or grow they slow.
>
> *(Ibid., p. 273)*

For Emerson and Thoreau, as with Blake before, the apparent boons promised by technology are ultimately empty and overshadowed by all that has been and will continue to be. One might observe the first stirrings of the ecological unconscious at Emerson and Thoreau's pond in Walden, just over a hundred years later Rachel Carson (1962) would publish her seminal environmental text 'Silent Spring'.

Carson's work exposed the dire ecological impact of the highly toxic pesticide/insecticide and persistent organic pollutant Dichlorodiphenyltrichloroethane (DDT). Whereas most insecticides of the day only targeted a couple of specific pests, DDT was far more potent, killing a great many more, much faster. But in our attempts to cheat or beat nature into producing ever higher crop yields, we were unconsciously, inadvertently poisoning our water, our soil, our ecosystem and ourselves. 'Silent Spring' convincingly and engagingly described the interconnectedness of all life and became a catalyst for the emergence of the Environmentalist movement. Carson's biophilia, her veneration of the natural world, clearly echoed that of both Emerson and Thoreau:

> Those who contemplate the beauty of the earth find reserves of strength that will endure as long as life lasts. There is something infinitely healing in the repeated refrains of nature – the assurance that dawn comes after night, and spring after winter.
>
> *(Carson 1998, p. 98)*

Sadly, what was once an *assurance* is now no longer so assured. Increasingly, weather forecasts report 'unseasonably' hot or cold weather, as extreme weather events become ever more frequent – enough to constitute a new normal. As the Anthropocene gathers speed, even the once comforting constant of the seasons is being challenged by climate change:

> The changing seasonal clock signifies disturbed agriculture seasons and rhythm of species activities, more frequent heat waves, storms and wildfires, amounting to increased risks to humanity.
>
> *(Wang et al. 2021, p. 1)*

There are even fears that if the world continues to warm, the season of Spring may eventually disappear entirely (Walsh 2014) – we may well be the generation that silenced Spring! What Lovelock (2009) once mourned as the 'Vanishing Face of Gaia' is experienced in real time, via the rapidly changing pace of nature. And if we continue to destroy our natural world, there will be no nature for us to rediscover and return to.

As technophilia rapidly overtakes biophilia and the Anthropocene is replaced by the Novacene (the new age of AI), we may begin to see ever less of ourselves reflected in the natural world, feeling ever more at home in our digital and virtual domains.

References

Alexander, C. (2004) *The Nature of Order: An Essay on Architecture and the Nature of the Universe: Part Four – The Luminous Ground*. Berkeley, CA: The Centre for Environmental Structure.

Alexander, C., Angel, S., Fiksdahl-King, I., Ishikawa, S., Silverstein, M. and Jacobson, M. (1977) *A Pattern Language*. Oxford: Oxford University Press.

Attenborough, D. (2019) Opening speech for Netflix series 'our planet'. *YouTube* [Online]. Available at: www.youtube.com/watch?v=X3stk6Gd5ss (Accessed 21 May 2023).

Björk (2011) *Biophilia*. London: One Little Indian.

Blake, W. (1982) *The Complete Poetry and Prose of William Blake: Newly Revised Edition* (Ed. Erdman, D.). Berkeley, CA: University of California Press.

Carson, R. (1962) *Silent Spring*. Boston, MA: Houghton Mifflin.

Carson, R. (1998) *The Sense of Wonder: A Celebration of Nature for Parents and Children*. New York: Harper Perennial.

Catton, W. and Dunlap, R. (1978) Environmental sociology: A new paradigm. *American Sociologist*, 13(1), pp. 11–19.

Cheney, I. (Director) (2011) *The City Dark* [Documentary]. New York: Rooftop Films and Edgeworx Studios.

Cohen, E. (2008) The tao of environmental psychology. *Transpersonal Psychology Review*, 12(2), pp. 32–38.

Cohen, N. and Eichenbaum, H. (1994) *Memory, Amnesia and the Hippocampal System*. Cambridge, MA: The MIT Press.

Douglass, P. (1986) *Bergson, Eliot and American Literature*. Lexington, KY: Kentucky University Press.

Emerson, R. W. (1995) *Essays and Poems*. London: Everyman.

French, H. T. and Rockwell, R. F. (2011) Climate change and avian population ecology in Europe. *Nature Education Knowledge*, 3(10), p. 1.

Fromm, E. (1973) *Anatomy of Human Destructiveness*. New York: Holt, Rinehart and Winston.

Gartner, C. (2017) Aristotle on love and friendship. In: Bobonich, C. (Ed.) *The* Cambridge *Companion to Ancient Ethics*. Cambridge: Cambridge University Press, pp. 143–162.

Hundertwasser, F. (1964) Mouldiness manifesto against rationalism in architecture. *Hundertwasser* [Online]. Available at: www.hundertwasser.at/english/texts/philo_verschimmelungsmanifest.php (Accessed 20 January 2023).

Hundertwasser, F. (1971) Forestation of the city. *Hundertwasser* [Online]. Available at: https://hundertwasser.com/en/texts/verwaldung_der_staedte (Accessed 20 January 2023).

Kaplan, R. and Kaplan, S. (1989) *The Experience of Nature: A Psychological Perspective*. Cambridge: Cambridge University Press.

Kellert, S., Heerwagen, J. and Mador, M. (2008) *Biophilic Design: The Theory, Science and Practice of Bringing Buildings to Life*. Hoboken, NJ: Wiley.

Kellert, S. and Wilson, E. (Eds.) (1993) *The Biophilia Hypothesis*. Washington, DC: Island Press.

Krause, B. (2012) *The Great Animal Orchestra: Finding the Origins of Music in the World's Wild Places*. London: Profile Books Limited.

Kunze, D., Brott, S. and Bertonlini, D. (Eds.) (2014) *Architecture Post Mortem: The Diastolic Architecture of Decline, Dystopia, and Death*. Oxon: Routledge.

Louv, R. (2005) *Last Child in the Woods: Saving Our Children from Nature Deficit Disorder*. Chapel Hill, NC: Algonquin Books.

Lovelock, J. (1979) *Gaia: A New Look at Life on Earth*. Oxford: Oxford University Press.

Lovelock, J. (2009) *The Vanishing Face of Gaia: A Final Warning*. London: Allen Lane.

Madden, D. (2022) Editorial – tired city: On the politics of urban exhaustion. *Analysis of Urban, Change, Theory, Action*, 26(4), pp. 559–561.

Naess, A. (1987) Self realisation: An ecological approach to being in the world. *The Trumpeter – Voices from the Canadian Ecophilosophy Net Work*, 4(3), pp. 35–42.

Posman, S. (2012) Time as a simple/multiple melody in Henri Bergson's "duration and simultaneity" and Gertrude Stein's landscape writing. *Mosaic: An Interdisciplinary Critical Journal*, 45(1), pp. 105–120.

Reilly, P. (1988) *The Lyrebird: A Natural History*. Sydney: New South Wales University Press.

Restany, P. (1998) *Hudertwasser: The Painter King with the Five Skins*. Glarus: Gruener Janura AG.

RHS (2023) Horatio's garden [Online]. Available at: www.rhs.org.uk/shows-events/rhs-chelsea-flower-show/Gardens/2023/horatios-garden (Accessed 20 January 2024).
Rosenblum, N. (Ed.) (2000) *Thoreau: Political Writings*. Cambridge: Cambridge University Press.
Roszak, T. (1992) *The Voice of the Earth: An Exploration of Ecopsychology*. New York: Simon & Schuster.
Sagan, C. (1980) *Cosmos* [Documentary Series]. Arlington: PBS.
Sagan, C. (2011) *The Pale Blue Dot: A Vision of the Human Future in Space*. New York: Random House Publishing.
Sturgeon, N. (1997) *Ecofeminist Natures: Race, Gender, Feminist Theory and Political Action*. Oxon: Routledge.
Snyder, G. (1969) *Smokey the bear sutra* [Online]. Available at: https://sacredtexts.com/bud/bear.htm (Accessed 21 May 2021).
Thoreau, H. D. (2004) *Walden and Other Writings*. New York: Bantam Dell.
Ulrich, R. S. (1984) View through a window may influence recovery from surgery. *Science*, 224(4647), pp. 420–421.
Walsh, B. (2014) The end of spring in a warming world. *Time* [Online]. Available at: https://time.com/30638/the-end-of-spring-in-a-warming-world/ (Accessed 21 May 2023).
Wang, J., Guan, Y., Wu, L., Guan, X., Cai, W., Huang, J., Dong, W. and Zhang, B. (2021) Changing lengths of the four seasons by global warming. *Geophysical Research Letters*, 48(6), pp. 1–9.
Winning, D. (2021) Astronomers can't hear signals from space because earth is too loud. *Wallstreet Journal* [Online]. Available at: www.wsj.com/articles/astronomers-cant-hear-signals-from-space-because-earth-is-too-loud-11615911902 (Accessed 21 May 2023).

6

STREAMS OF CONSCIOUSNESS, STREAMS OF DATA

The Sinclair ZX Spectrum 48K was our family's very first computer. Designed by Sir Clive Sinclair (1940–2021), a pioneer in consumer electronics and home computing, it was launched with great fanfare in 1982. I can still vividly recollect its rainbow logo and distinctive rubber keys. This was the first machine I ever learnt to program in order to write my own games. Although these were admittedly very basic games with crude graphics accompanied by 1-bit soundtracks, the ability to construct virtual worlds, wherein I would be the one to set the parameters and populate with my own digital creations was an early and intoxicating taste of omnipotence or cyberpotence.

The inordinate amount of time I spent indoors programming as opposed to playing outdoors was occasionally a matter of concern for my parents, but there remained the hope that I was acquiring important, transferable skills. Seymour Papert, an influential South-African-American mathematician, computer scientist and the 'father of educational computing' (Stager 2016) enthusiastically promoted computers as a tool to enhance children's learning. 'In Papert's eyes, the computer was an object to think with' (Ibid.).

> In many schools today, the phrase 'computer-aided instruction' means making the computer teach the child. One might say the computer is being used to program the child. In my vision, the child programs the computer and, in doing so, both acquires a sense of mastery over a piece of the most modern and powerful technology and establishes an intimate contact with some of the deepest ideas from science, from mathematics, and from the art of intellectual model building.
>
> *(Papert 1980, p. 5)*

DOI: 10.4324/9781003334972-6

More recently, it appears that the computer has increasingly become an object to emulate and think *like*.

Computational Thinking formally became part of the UK's Computing National Curriculum in 2014, emphasising the core skills of algorithmic thinking, decomposition, generalisation, abstraction and evaluation (Csizmadia et al. 2015). Today, it is not simply regarded as a useful skill but is seen by many as 'the fundamental skill for scientific, technological and economic development for the twenty-first century' (Belmar 2022).

I remain unconvinced that my many hundreds of hours spent programming the ZX Spectrum instilled or enabled a more computational outlook on my world. Aside from the occasional, fleeting sensation of mastery, my cognitive style was, and remains, rather more intuitive and heuristic rather than systematic and algorithmic. One might also consider that the computer I was using was, from a contemporary standpoint, very basic.

By today's technological standards, in our new age of accelerated computing, the 48K ZX Spectrum is a technological relic. Even the small, sleek mobile phone tucked snugly into my jacket pocket is thousands of times more powerful and faster than my first computer.

The mobile phone is a familiar example of the ongoing trend towards miniaturisation and ephermeralisation. The American architect and futurist Richard Buckminster Fuller famously predicted (in 1938) that technological advancement will allow us to 'do more and more with less and less until eventually you can do everything with nothing' (quoted in Southerton 2011, p. 433). Indeed, our world appears to be dematerialising before us, becoming less and less substantial. Whereas once my home was filled with records, tapes, CDs, books and photo albums, now each and every one of these can easily fit inside my phone with space to spare.

Because it does and contains so much, the mobile phone now occupies a uniquely central place in our modern lives. To be separated from one's phone can elicit a genuine sense of anxiety amongst many people, leading to the emergence of a very contemporary condition 'Nomophobia' – referring to No Mobile Phobia (Bhattacharya et al. 2019). Although Nomphobia is usually discussed more generally within the clinical contexts of anxiety and digital addiction, I believe it is better understood in relation to the mobile phone's increased incorporation into our self-concept. Our phones both contain and connect us to so much of what we identify *as* and *with* that they have become, in quite a short period of time, not merely extensions of ourselves but integral parts of ourselves.

In 1984 (only one year after the official birthday of the internet), the American Sociologist Sherry Turkle had begun to explore our relationship with the world of computing and identified the emergence of a so-called 'Second Self' (Turkle 2005). Turkle observed and ably analysed the manner in which technology had rapidly transformed from something external to us and essentially alien, into something altogether more intimate. This intimacy intensifies as a result of both our increasing familiarity with the digital domain and the technological advancements that make this domain ever more present and immersive.

More recently, entrepreneur and futurist Elon Musk has been developing and promoting technologies such as *Neuralink* – brain–computer interfaces. One mainstream media headline reported that we were already witnessing the 'Dawn of the Cyborg' (Hooper 2024) as 'Musk puts first chip in Human brain' (Ibid.).

In a short time, it may become increasingly difficult to determine where we end, and our machines begin. It no longer appears to be such a dramatic leap from wearable technology to integrated technology, cybernetic enhancements and upgrades:

> We already have a digital tertiary layer in a sense, in that you have your computer or your phone or your applications . . . The thing that people, I think, don't appreciate right now is that they are already a cyborg . . . If you leave your phone behind, it's like missing limb syndrome. I think people – they're already kind of merged with their phone and their laptop and their applications and everything.
>
> *(Musk quoted in Houser 2017)*

Or as the comedian Jerry Seinfeld insightfully quipped:

> That's why it's called an iPhone, it's half myself, half phone – that's a complete individual!
>
> *(Seinfeld 2020)*

In respect to our technologies, we appear to have evolved from being simply *users* to *fusers*. To adapt or update Erich Fromm's terminology, we might say technology has shifted from something *to have* to opening new frontiers of *being*. As we continue to move beyond using technology and increasingly fusing with it, our conversation inevitably shifts from human nature to Transhuman nature.

Popular TV series such as 'Black Mirror' (2011–ongoing) often explore or exploit our dystopian fears and fantasies concerning such a transhuman future. We may never have been truly able to pass through the looking glass, but we appear daily ever closer to passing through the computer monitor – inhabiting and exploring more virtual realms and realities. We can immerse ourselves in digital realms of virtual reality, or else the digital realm may seemingly extend outwards towards us in the form of augmented realities, where virtual worlds are superimposed upon our physical world. The computer monitor appears ever less like a display and ever more as a portal.

Even the need for a physical computer monitor may itself soon seem antiquated, as technological advancements continue to gather pace and screens continue to become slimmer and less substantial – recent developments now include augmented reality displays. What was once the latest innovation can quickly slip into antiquation – and we may find ourselves struggling to keep up with the latest technological trends. In this sense perhaps we never succeed in escaping the mode of having, and we remain consumers before fusers. But for all our apparent intense dependence on and attachment to our mobile phones, this dependence appears quite malleable and transferable whenever a newer, superior model appears.

The constant arrival of state-of-the-art, new and improved mobile phones, much-anticipated product unveilings and launches, has all the hallmarks of dynamic obsolescence – an implicit admission and recognition that all things are 'made to break' (Slade 2009). One cannot help but wonder if integration and enhancement become the norm, will transhumans also be made to break, and thus forced into a life of perpetual purchasing, enhancing, and upgrading. In 1928, Herbert Hoover, only months prior to being elected President of the United States, had lavished praise upon the early architects of advertising and public relations (including Freud's nephew Edward Bernays) who conceived much of what has become our familiar consumer culture, in terms which now seem eerily prophetic:

> You have taken over the job of creating desire and have transformed people into constantly moving happiness machines. Machines which have become the key to economic progress.
>
> *(Hoover quoted in Saxena 2021, p. 119)*

But the mindset of constant consumption, our 'cultures of excess' (Slosar 2009), arguably produce less lasting happiness than they do a great deal of waste that is difficult to dispose of.

The journey from new, top-of-the-line, 'must have' purchase to outdated, disposable, bottom-of-the-heap refuse is increasingly short. The growing number of 'manufactured landscapes' (Baichwal 2008), the rising mountains and valleys of e-waste captured in the industrial landscape photography of Canadian artist Edward Burtynsky, is a shocking illustration of the problem. Baichwal's documentary/horror depicts a disconcerting future where we appear to be drowning in our own waste. But the production line never seems to stop, the machines making the machines neither sleep nor slow down.

The sheer pace of change appears to be outrunning, overtaking and obsoleting the very models designed to measure the pace of change. For almost sixty years, Moore's law accurately predicted that processing power of computers would double every couple of years; an acceleration due to the doubling number of transistors in an integrated circuit. More recent discussions and debates concerning 'accelerating change' describe an exponential rise in technological advancement that we cannot yet begin to fathom, let alone accurately predict or adequately prepare for. Ray Kurzweil, an American computer scientist and futurist, outlined his law of accelerating returns in terms that appear to intentionally blur the lines between science fiction and science fact:

> An analysis of the history of technology shows that technological change is exponential, contrary to the common-sense 'intuitive linear' view. So we won't experience 100 years of progress in the 21st century – it will be more like 20,000 years of progress (at today's rate). The 'returns,' such as chip speed and cost-effectiveness, also increase exponentially. There's even exponential growth in the rate of exponential growth. Within a few decades, machine intelligence will surpass human intelligence, leading to the Singularity – technological change so rapid and profound it represents a rupture in the fabric of human history. The implications include the merger of biological and nonbiological intelligence, immortal software-based humans, and ultra-high levels of intelligence that expand outward in the universe at the speed of light.
>
> *(Kurzweil quoted in Cordeiro 2019, p. 66)*

Where and What Are We?

In our Social Psychology degree at Leeds Beckett University, we begin our second year's Environmental Psychology module by considering 'Space and Place'. The very first question the students are asked and required to answer by way of illustration and personal reflection is 'Where are you right now?'

Most students respond by drawing their position in the classroom, sketching their desk in spatial relation to other desks, or broadening the scale to include the various campus buildings in relation to significant Leeds landmarks, the Rose Bowl or Parkinson Tower. Some students interpret the question less geographically, spatially and more psychologically – reflecting on their emotional state or what is presently foremost on their mind as being *where* they currently are. One mature student once admitted that although appearing to be physically present, they were mentally in Paris, replaying and reliving a recent holiday with their partner. Increasingly, students are also recognising how, whilst seemingly simply sitting in a classroom, they are simultaneously inhabiting multiple virtual spaces by virtue of their online presence/s – often consisting of several virtual selves, digitally dispersed across various social networking sites and online platforms – constituting a virtual omnipresence. In this way, the question 'Where are you?' leads directly to a deeper ontological question 'What are you?'

Environmental Psychology has furnished us with relatable theories explaining how place continually shapes our sense of sense. When we casually ask a person 'Where are you from?', implicit in this line of questioning is the belief that knowing the location of their upbringing will provide some helpful contextual clues about their character and perhaps some insight into their background and lived experience.

Place Attachment Theory observes how we may be deeply drawn to certain places, so much so that we may psychologically and emotionally internalise them forming a place identity (Gifford 2014). People from big cities such as New York or London may be assumed to possess a more urban psyche. New York, in particular, is often said to be a 'state of mind' as much as it is a physical place. The corresponding New York personality is famously fast, has no time for nonsense and is fiercely independent, outspoken and abrupt. The sheer speed, size and complexity of such megacities can be disorientating and overwhelming. My first time in Tokyo Japan was one such experience – the sheer density of hurrying humanity, the perpetually flashing neon signs and competing digital displays, and the constant cries of department store greeters (some human, some mechanised) battling against the deafening blare of pachinko parlours.

The topophobia I experienced in Tokyo was equalled by the restorative topophilia I encountered in Kyoto with its charming character-filled, lantern-lit cobblestone streets, and warm and welcoming *machiya*-style wooden temples and tea houses. Kyoto is justifiably famed for its preservation of traditional Japanese culture. Curiously, modern Japan is celebrated as much for its artistic and cultural heritage as it is known for its embrace of technology, particularly robotics – indeed their apparent harmonious coexistence, this happy marriage between the past and the future, can be a source of puzzlement to many Westerners.

Part of this harmony may be due to familiarity. Whereas in the West we may perceive the attempts of designers and manufacturers to make robots appear more human as disturbing or uncanny, in Japan they appear to be more widely and readily accepted and embraced, as explored in Hornyak's (2006) 'Loving the Machine'. In more recent times, this 'loving' relationship has intensified into a more devotional dynamic as robots begin to take a more central role in some Buddhist temples. Robots have been designed that can chant Buddhist sutras at funeral services and some have even been modelled to resemble Buddhist deities.

In Kyoto's historic Zen Buddhist temple *Kodaiji*, one can now receive Dharma teachings and blessings from Mindar, the world's first robotic Bodhisattva (originally installed in 2019). Whilst Mindar's body comprises of cold, bare aluminium, the silicone face appears far more lifelike, modelled on the popular Buddhist deity Kannon, the Bodhisattva of Infinite Compassion. The abbot of the temple, Tensho Goto, had hoped that this innovative inclusion of cutting-edge technology, robotics allied with artificial intelligence (AI), might succeed in revolutionising and renewing Buddhism in Japan whilst also attracting more of the younger generation to the temple.

A central principle in Mahayana Buddhism is *Upaya-kaushalya* or skilful means, referring to the way one creatively adapts and tailors one's teachings to be more intelligible and relatable to one's audience. In Japan Kanon appears as a male deity, but in China they preferred and more readily revered a female form for the embodiment of compassion, which is why one typically finds the Goddess Guan Yin in most Chinese Buddhist temples. Both Kanon and Guan Yin were local adaptations of the original Indian Bodhisattva called Avalokitesvara (a name which means 'to look down upon with compassion'). Avalokitesvara appears infinitely adaptable – sometimes appearing in recognisably human form, perhaps disguised as a beggar or even a queen – other times transforming into a more cosmic manifestation, spontaneously sprouting one thousand arms in order to reach out to all suffering sentient beings – a striking visual embodiment of *Upaya*.

One might also consider the Dalai Lama's enthusiastic embrace of the natural sciences, particularly physics and neuroscience, as a similar example of skilful means, that allows him to more easily connect to and communicate with Western audiences – translating the ancient Buddhist religion into a contemporary mind science. It is significant to recall that the Dalai Lama is also viewed by Tibetan Buddhists as a living incarnation of Avalokitesvara, called Chenrezig in Tibetan. When one considers the prevalence and popularity of technology (particularly robotics) in Japan, Tensho Goto's decision to install Mindar seems quite pragmatic, serving as a bridge between the traditional and the modern:

> Artificial intelligence has developed to such an extent we thought it logical for the Buddha to transform into a robot.
>
> *(Tensho Goto quoted in Himmer 2019)*

The abbot initially noted that the only real resistance appeared to come from Western visitors who perceived Mindar as more of a barrier than a bridge, comparing it to 'Frankenstein's monster' (Ibid.). Similar sentiments had been explored earlier in Mim's (2010) paper published in the *MIT Technology Review* 'Why Japanese Love Robots (and Americans Fear Them)':

> Japanese culture predisposes its members to look at robots as helpmates and equals imbued with something akin to the Western conception of a soul, while Americans view robots as dangerous and willful constructs who will eventually bring about the death of their makers.
>
> *(Ibid.)*

To date, there have been several collective, but largely unheeded calls to slow down or pause the development of ever more powerful generative AI before we have had time to properly consider the potential consequences. One popular petition launched by the *Future of Life Institute* (2023) contained questions which raised alarming apocalyptic scenarios:

> Should we develop nonhuman minds that might eventually outnumber, outsmart, obsolete and replace us? Should we risk loss of control of our civilization?
>
> *(Ibid.)*

In the same year, a celebrated pioneer of AI, the Cognitive Psychologist Geoffrey Hinton, resigned from Google due to his fears concerning the ongoing and unchecked military deployment of Artificial Intelligence. A familiar expression one might encounter is that, regarding AI, the 'genie is already out of the bottle'. But perhaps it might be more appropriate to say that 'the golem is already out of the attic'.

The golem of legend is an artificial life form, composed of clay and animated by secret Divine names. The most famous story of golem remains that of the Rabbi Judah Loew's (1525–1609 CE) golem of Prague, constructed to protect the oft-persecuted Jewish community. When not engaged in defending the community, the golem would complete simple, mundane tasks, often in a manner which displayed his superhuman strength and speed – one example includes the Rabbi's wife requesting the golem to fetch water from the local well, which soon leads to the whole home and street being flooded. Similar tales relate to Rabbi Elijah of Chelm in the sixteenth century who also created a golem but:

> When the creature attained giant size and strength, the Rabbi, appalled by its destructive potentialities, tore the life giving name from its forehead and it crumbled into dust.
>
> *(Trachtenberg 2004, p. 85)*

Trachtenberg observes how these stories appear as forerunners to the more famous gothic horror of Frankenstein's monster – with its central theme of playing God. In more recent permutations of the tale, the golem becomes a precursor of artificial intelligence. In one particularly curious article, Mitchell Marcus (1999) notes that three of the founding figures of Artificial Intelligence at MIT – Joel Moses, Gerry Sussman and Marvin Minsky – not only shared a Jewish heritage but were also each reputedly a direct descendent of Rabbi Judah Loew. Marcus even quotes Sussman, making the lineage more explicit – 'You know, we computer scientists are really the Kabbalists of today. We animate these inanimate machines by getting strings of symbols just right' (Ibid., p. 370).

Both the jinn or golems of folklore appear to have much in common with the existential threats many leading scientists and technologists fear may await us in the near future.

One recent film that vividly reflected these fears was 'The Creator' (Edwards 2023), where AI is (mistakenly) blamed, and subsequently banned, for initiating a nuclear war against humanity. A costly conflict ensues between humanity and AI, which escalates into a global struggle between the AI-phobic West (primarily America) and the AI-philic East, set in the year 2050. The film's fictional depiction of the East's embrace of technology also includes a significant devotional dimension. Robotic beings are frequently presented in the familiar saffron robes of Buddhist monks, guarding a being named *Nimrata* (the Sanskrit term for creator) whose human name is *Maya* (a Sanskrit word meaning illusion, but which is also the name of the historical Buddha's mother). The futuristic transhuman neo-Buddhist iconography displayed in the temple scenes towards the end of the movie is uncannily reminiscent of Mindar. For the present, however, it appears Mindar may not be replacing the human monks of Kodaiji Temple.

More recent findings from the *Scientific American* suggest that devotees are not particularly moved or inspired by the machine, due to a lack of perceived 'credibility' (Jackson and Yam 2023). Mindar may chant flawlessly, but it does not and cannot truly understand the significance of anything it is chanting. Mindar may preach convincingly about compassion but is not capable of feeling it. Conversely, one might argue that Mindar is also entirely free from anger and craving, two of the traditional three poisons that prevent us from achieving Buddhahood, but admittedly this is all by design – for Mindar nothing has been truly attained.

Aside from serving as a curiosity, Mindar doesn't appear to be attracting significantly more people into the temple. As less people were physically visiting the temples, due to the frantic pace of life coupled with waning interest in religion, there had been an earlier attempt to respond to this by moving some temples and pilgrimage centres online. These more virtual forms of veneration were termed *Ea Sampai* エア参拝 or 'Air Worship'. Similarly, during the global pandemic, devotees of the international *Fo Guang Shan* Buddhist fellowship were instead invited to bathe the virtual body of the Buddha at the movement's website, rather than physically gathering at the temple to conduct the ceremony that traditionally marks the Buddha's birth and awakening.

Unable to leave the house during lockdown, many new and innovative forms of 'virtual tourism' (Cheng and Huang 2022) became and remain far more commonplace. Irrespective of one's technophilic or technophobic predilections, it is difficult to deny that the internet is radically transforming both our sense of space and place and our sense of self.

The various home pages we visit daily may indeed appear increasingly homely, familiar, and welcoming. One might even note that as our physical built environments appear to have become ever more homogenous, sterile *spaces*, by contrast, our digital domains become ever more humanised, personalised *places*. Part of this may be accounted for due to the fact that instrumental software engineers such as Kent Beck and Ward Cunningham, founders of the pattern movement, were directly influenced by the architectural work of Christopher Alexander and sought to apply it to user interfaces in the 1980s (Ghidersa 2022).

Whenever I visit Facebook, X (formerly Twitter), Instagram, etc., I find I am able to quite easily navigate or wayfind through the websites. I am also encouraged to create and personalise my profile until it reflects either an imagined real or ideal virtual version of my self-concept. I may then begin to form connections with individuals and groups that both reflect, reinforce and expand my social identity. It is far from uncommon to find oneself becoming increasingly immersed and invested in these online identities, places and communities – as it is particularly easy to lose track of screen time, the Covid epidemic only served to further amplify and embed this effect.

John R. Suler (2016), one of the early pioneers of Cyberpsychology, discussed these themes of time, place and identity in his 'Psychology of the Digital Age: Humans Become Electric'. One example that Suler repeatedly returns to and reflects on is his personal time spent in the graphical chat room called The Palace. The Palace consisted of various virtual rooms where customised avatars could interact via speech bubbles containing written text. Based on the richness of his ethnographic reflections and psychoanalytic interpretations, Suler undoubtedly spent a great deal of time in the Palace. When introducing the 'architecture' of cyberpsychology, he notes the experience of 'accelerated time':

> Time in cyberspace can feel accelerated, in part due to the fact that online environments change rapidly.
>
> *(Ibid., p. 43)*

I have also noted vocal resistance to change, particularly when websites seek to update, redesign or reinvent themselves. On several occasions, over fifteen years of membership, I have observed Facebook users consistently voice distress or disapproval whenever a new page layout is proposed or applied. Following the flurry of complaints about 'change for change's sake', there typically follow posts linking to online tutorials instructing users how to recover the more familiar and comforting 'classic' layout. It appears quite evident that there have emerged novel forms of virtual place attachment and identity. This becomes even clearer and seemingly inevitable when one considers our increasingly excessive time spent online set alongside the role duration or length of association plays in establishing, strengthening and deepening our attachment to place. It has become far less of a cyberspace and more of a cyberplace.

Virtual and augmented realities continue to make the distance and difference between the physical and the virtual appear ever more permeable and traversable. As technologies such as Neurolink become ever more advanced and accessible, we may soon inhabit these digital realms as naturally as we currently inhabit our physical realm – consequently, the very meanings of natural and nature may change. Our expanding universe has been joined by the expanding metaverse. Richard Louv lamented the 'Last Child in Woods' (2005), and in time we come to witness the first child in the machine.

Speaking and Thinking Like a Machine

> We create tools and then we mold ourselves in their image. Seventeenth-century clockworks inspired mechanistic metaphors ('The heart is a pump'), just as the self-regulating engineering devices of the mid-twentieth century inspired the cybernetic image ('The brain is a computer').
>
> (Brockman 2010)

Today, one cannot help but notice the increasing ubiquity and dominance of digital discourse. Turkle (2005) had previously noted the emergence and proliferation of digital discursive trends as early as the 1970s and 1980s:

> people in their everyday conversation began to describe human mental activity in computational terms. ('Excuse me, I need to clear my buffer; I won't be happy until I debug this problem.')
>
> *(Turkle 2005, p. 2)*

It is still not uncommon to hear reference to people, habits and behaviours being 'hardwired', relating to and reimagining our biology as a form of hardware or software. This deterministic language is still quite regularly encountered in popular sayings such as 'neurons that fire together wire together'.

When Barrett and Francescutti (2020) discuss the deteriorating health and diminishing lifespans of Americans, paradoxically in the midst of an information age, where we have more access to medical- and health-related knowledge than at any other time in human history, they identify our evolutionary 'hardwiring' as one of the main culprits. When considering the compelling, addictive nature of social media, they observe:

> In our own hardwired brains, we also produce our own in-house 'drugs,' in the forms of neurotransmitters that feed voraciously off social status. To be liked and admired by others, to feel belonging and to garner sexual

> attention are eternally sparking survival instincts upon which social media pours pure gasoline. While we all possess this hardwired software, most of us never realise that it is running in the background, controlling our moods and behaviour.
>
> *(p. xi)*

During my time as a Psychology undergraduate (1997–2000), the language was already shifting from describing the brain as being hardwired to instead emphasising its plasticity, specifically neuroplasticity. The resultant atmosphere and outlook were arguably more optimistic, as our inherent capacity to grow and change was more commonly emphasised. We were in fact warned by our lecturers that to refer to either the brain or human behaviour as 'hardwired' was anachronistic, and that we may consequently lose marks in our neuropsychology assignments. One can certainly appreciate how if the brain and behaviour were fixed in the sense of being hardwired it would potentially render much of psychology (in general) and psychotherapy (in particular), as primarily descriptive disciplines, reducing their capacity for meaningful transformation.

In contemporary forms of Neuroscience, Cognitive Psychology and Cognitive Behavioural Therapy (CBT), technological terminology and digital discourse abound. The brain is often described and related to in terms of neural networks and cortical circuitry. Cognitive Psychology, with its various models of memory and attention, typically re-renders the human being as an information processor.

Mainstream cognitive models of depression emulate computational thinking and adopt the increasingly familiar form of algorithmic flowcharts. In Figure 6.1, we see an illustration of 'information processing in the cognitive model of depression' (Disner et al. 2011, p. 469) published in the journal *Nature Reviews*.

My once familiar thoughts and feelings are now reconfigured as schema activation that may result in biased processing.

In one popular clinical example, the experience of not being acknowledged by a friend passing in the street serves to demonstrate the potentially pernicious cycles of distorted thinking. Perhaps an underlying mechanism of low self-esteem may more easily lead to, or *activate* the perception of 'I'm being ignored', with all the related ruminations of self-blame – 'Why are they angry with me? What did I do wrong?' Once I encounter this environmental trigger, my schemas are activated. This, in turn, may result in a proliferation of negative automatic thoughts (NATs), for example, 'I am a bad friend. I am always upsetting people.' I continue to process the encounter in a bias manner, which in turn only serves to further reinforce my depressive symptoms. Perhaps some hours after the encounter, I am still replaying the events, alongside the associated hurt, self-critical thoughts, and recollections of comparable,

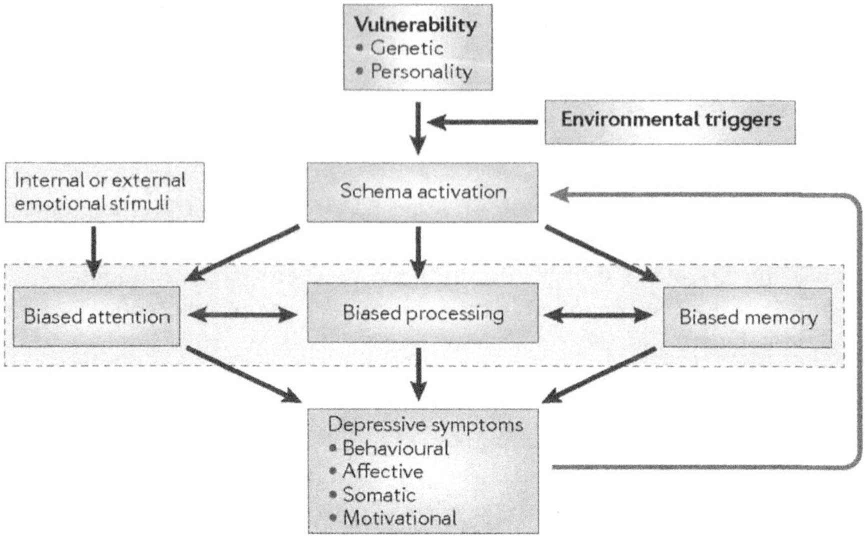

FIGURE 6.1 Information processing in the cognitive model of depression (Disner et al. 2011, p. 469)

historical, painful or awkward encounters – seemingly trapped in a ruminative feedback loop. In my quieter, more introspective moments, my thoughts and feelings may continue to intrude and disrupt my well-being.

Neuroscientists studying the neural correlates of consciousness (NCCs) propose that an interconnected group of brain structures termed the Default Mode Network (DMN), which are primarily related to the wandering mind, imagination and introspection, may in such cases be overactive (Ramirez 2015). This excessive activity occurring within the DMN may itself be due to a form of miswiring, more technically termed abnormal functional connectivity within the neural network.

By contrast, my focused, directed and attentive mind may be termed the Task-Positive Network (TPN) and is related to my Executive Function (EF). Recent Third Wave Cognitive Therapies that utilise Mindfulness-Based Approaches will commonly list the positive effects of meditation as including reduced activity within the Default Mode Network, and alternately supporting and enhancing Executive Function.

With the advent of increasingly sophisticated brain imaging technology, the meditator's brain may now be studied and measured. At the *Mind and Life Institute*, where neuroscientists have been collaborating with contemplatives since 1987, experienced meditators are frequently connected to Electro Encephalograph (EEG) machines to measure their cortical oscillations during varied, deep states of meditative activity and absorption. During much of our daily activity, our default brainwave remains around the Beta frequency band. More relaxed states are correlated with Alpha states, and these are also often associated with more mindful types of attention.

In November 2012, the *Smithsonian Magazine* declared that they had located 'the world's happiest man' (Nuwer 2012). The headline read that 'Matthieu Ricard, a 66-year-old Tibetan monk and geneticist, produces brain gamma waves never before reported in neuroscience' (Ibid.). Ricard himself modestly dismissed these claims and declared this headline to be 'the biggest joke in the world' (Ricard 2023, p. 578). However, new neurofeedback techniques continue to promote the possibility of retraining the brain, allowing more people to access meditative states without the years of intensive training and retreats. When addressing the Annual Meeting of the Society for Neuroscience in Washington in 2005, the Dalai Lama had reiterated his admiration for science and technology, and proceeded to remark that should neuroscientists start to develop technologies which would allow people to access meditative states without the time-demanding and often arduous effort required, he would offer himself up as enthusiastic experimental subject (Reiner 2009).

Only three years after this meeting, I had been introduced to a new contemplative technology called *Holosync*®, at the first international Integral Theory Conference in California in 2008. Integral Theory was the brainchild of the philosopher Ken Wilber, who had previously demonstrated his own meditative virtuosity in a popular video published by *Integral Life* titled 'Ken Wilber Stops His Brainwaves' (Integral Life 2006). In this video, Wilber seemingly, voluntarily reduces all his measurable brain activity, as measured on a small portable EEG machine, through engaging in various types of advanced, formless meditation. This ability to consciously manipulate his cortical oscillations was largely the result of many decades of engagement with and immersion in various contemplative disciplines. A more popular estimate suggests that 10,000 hours of practice typically leads to expertise in any activity from musicianship to meditation, and this level or duration of experience is usually required for someone to be considered an experienced meditator in psychological research. The *Holoysnc*® technology initially caught my attention due to its particularly bold tagline:

> with The *Holosync*® Solution, you'll *meditate deeper than a Zen Monk* at the push of a button.
>
> *(Centrepointe 2024)*

Continuing:

> Using powerful, proprietary brainwave technology, Holosync strengthens the 'executive function' (willpower, focus, creativity) of your brain, while it calms the areas that create stress, impulsive behaviors and procrastination.
>
> *(Ibid.)*

As a longtime meditator I was intrigued, whilst simultaneously harbouring profound reservations, concerning this rather incredulous-sounding claim. Nevertheless, I signed up for the workshop.

We were provided with soft seating and large comfortable headphones and told to sit still and simply listen. What soon followed was the soothing sound of white noise, occasionally punctuated with deep, resonant chimes occurring in different ears. My reflective notes from the session read 'like attending a gamelan concert in the pouring rain'. Although undoubtedly relaxing and restorative, I would not necessarily have described the activity as deep meditation – there was nothing approaching the deep absorption of the Jhanas or any glimpse of awakening, neither *kensho* nor *satori*. In fairness, this was my first attempt at using the technology, but to be equally fair I had been assured the results of many years' practice instantaneously – 'at the push of a button'.

It is worth reflecting that patience and persistence are both included in the traditional Buddhist list of the Six Perfections, as integral qualities that precede and support meditation. A popular Zen tale illustrates this point, describing an impatient student asking his master how long it will take for him to reach enlightenment. The master silently examines the student for some time and eventually replies 'From where you are now – about ten years'. The student appears disconcerted, exclaiming 'That's far too long! What about if I was to spend every minute of every day practicing with you for the next few years?' The master pauses and replies 'From where you are right now – about twenty years!' This counter-intuitive Zen teaching encourages us to focus more on the *process* and *practice* of meditation rather than becoming fixated on outcomes or time-saving strategies.

But if the mind *is* essentially machine-like, akin to a sophisticated computer program, why couldn't or shouldn't it be hacked? Both the term and activity of hacking still retain or evoke troubling elements of ethical ambiguity or even criminality. One may hack into a system in order to steal personal data, with the nefarious intention of committing fraud or identity theft. One may hack into a computer game in order to gain an unearned and unfair advantage over other players, receiving rewards or even skipping entire levels – in this sense, the hack is synonymous with cheat codes or exploits.

Terms such as 'life hacks' and 'mind hacks' have indeed become increasingly commonplace, promising time-saving shortcuts that will allow us to circumvent extensive effort, do away with the need for patience, and enable us to achieve our desires ever more efficiently and rapidly. Concurrent with the digital age, alongside the novel, alluring descriptions of neural networks appeared the Promethean promise that one might be able to hack into the source code of the psyche, to reprogram the mind or rewire the brain.

The idea of working for or towards one's happiness may begin to sound increasingly archaic, as more reductionist and machine-like models of mind become ever more popular and prevalent. The mind and brain both become reconfigured in a manner which gives primary importance to and emphasis on internal reward systems, and explanations concerning how to quickly and easily locate and activate one's hedonic hotspots. The dopaminergic mesolimbic system is frequently mentioned as being one of the dominant reward pathways in the brain, and many popular online articles will list numerous simple activities intended to lead to a rapid release or 'rush' of Dopamine, eliciting a strong sense of satisfaction and achievement.

Implicit in this 'mind hacking' is the unstated principle that the ends are ultimately more important than the means, and that happiness, love, self-worth, and sense of achievement are all in essence neurochemical, capable of being manufactured by mechanical means.

As the model of the mechanised mind becomes more familiar and continues to gain currency, both psychology and psychotherapy may become increasingly akin to mapping, identifying and correcting our psychological source code – consequently, psychotherapists may increasingly transform into technicians:

> The recent and rapid rise of online, virtual e-therapies and increasing experimentation with non-human, automated therapists (evidenced in the proliferation of 'therapy apps') is another worrying part of this overall trend towards artificiality and algocracy. This trend may become ever more entrenched if we continue to internalize this more mechanized view of the mind – for if we are ultimately understood to be algorithmic at our very core, then what better than an algorithm to treat us or even eventually lead us?
>
> *(Cohen 2024, p. 109)*

James Lovelock's (2019) final book 'Novacene' was a surprisingly optimistic ode to our future, hyperintelligent AI overlords. Rather than viewing our future as a one of fusing with our machines, Lovelock saw our role as the parents or midwives to an entirely new and arguably far superior form of life. These living AI machines may be a million times faster than us (Ibid., p. 81) – subsequently their thought processes and forms of communication may be utterly incomprehensible to us. One consequence of this is that, compared to these machines, we may appear as slow and incommunicative as plants:

> The experience of watching your garden grow gives you some idea of how future AI systems will feel when observing human life.
>
> *(Ibid., pp. 81–82)*

In contrast to the popular humanoid depictions of AI robots, Lovelock imagines sphere-like beings that may be both unimaginably fast and small, with reality-bending implications:

> The speed and power of their thoughts will give them access to the mysteries that baffle us, such as the apparent ability of particles to send signals faster than the speed of light and to be in two places at once, and many more.
>
> *(Ibid., p. 102)*

Lovelock's optimism reached a crescendo in Chapter 20 – 'All Watched Over by Machines of Loving Grace' (Ibid., p. 104), when he proposed that the AI life forms we produce will likely look upon us, their primitive biological forebears, with benevolence.

In the end, perhaps it will not be *we* who grow through our machines, but rather our machines which ultimately outgrow *us*. Whilst these AI life forms explore new world systems, dimensions and quantum realms we would struggle to conceive of, humanity may inadvertently find ourselves brought back down to Earth – back to the garden, where it all began.

References

Baichwal, J. (Dir.) (2008) *Manufactured Landscapes*. Mercury Films Inc. and Foundry Films Inc. in Co-production with the National Film Board of Canada and in Association with TV Ontario. Quebec, Montreal.

Barrett, R. and Francescutti, H. (2020) *Hardwired: How Our Instincts to Be Healthy Are Making Us Sick*. New York: Springer.

Belmar, H. (2022) Review on the teaching of computer programming and computational thinking in the world. *Frontiers in Computer Science*, 4. Available at: www.frontiersin.org/articles/10.3389/fcomp.2022.997222/full

Bhattacharya, S., Bashar, M. A., Srivastava, A. and Singh, A. (2019) NOMOPHOBIA: NO MObile PHone PhoBIA. *Journal of Family Medicine and Primary Care*, 8(4), pp. 1297–1300.

Black Mirror (2011–ongoing) *Series 1–6* [Streaming Series]. Los Gatos, CA: Netflix.

Brockman, J. (2010) The edge annual question 2010: How is the Internet changing the way you think? [Online]. Available at: www.huffpost.com/entry/the-collective-conscious_b_418453 (Accessed 8 March 2024).

Centrepointe (2024) What is holosync? [Online]. Available at: www.centerpointe.com/what-is-holosync/ (Accessed 10 April 2024).

Cheng, L. K. and Huang, H. L. (2022) Virtual tourism atmospheres: The effects of pleasure, arousal, and dominance on the acceptance of virtual tourism. *Journal of Hospitality and Tourism Management*, 53, pp. 143–152.

Cohen, E. (2024) The dao of dialogue: Daoism, psychology and psychotherapy. *Journal of Daoist Studies*, 17, pp. 99–116.

Cordeiro, J. L. (2019) The boundaries of the human: From human to transhuman. In: Lee, N. (Ed.) *The Transhuman Handbook*. New York: Springer, pp. 63–74.

Csizmadia, A., Curzon, P., Dorling, M., Humphreys, S., Ng, T., Selby, C. and Woollard, J. (2015) *Computational Thinking: A Guide for Teachers*. Swindon: Computing at School.

Disner, S., Beevers, C., Haigh, E. and Beck, A. (2011) Neural mechanisms of the cognitive model of depression. *Nature Reviews Neuroscience*, 12, pp. 467–477.
Edwards, G. (Dir.) (2023) *The Creator*. Los Angeles, CA: 20th Century Studios.
Future of Life Institute (2023) Pause giant AI experiments: An open letter [Online]. Available at: https://futureoflife.org/open-letter/pause-giant-ai-experiments/ (Accessed 25 March 2023).
Ghidersa, M. R. (2022) *Software Architecture for Web Developers*. Birmingham: Packt Publishing Ltd.
Gifford, R. (2014) *Environmental Psychology: Principles and Practice*. Boston, MA: Allyn and Bacon.
Himmer, A. (2019) Japan times [Online]. Available at: www.japantimes.co.jp/news/2019/08/15/business/tech/kyoto-temple-robot-priest/#.XvyGY-fTXIU (Accessed 1 July 2020).
Hooper, S. (2024) Dawn of the cyborg. *MetroUK* [Online]. Available at: https://twitter.com/MetroUK/status/1752437868927025274
Hornyak, T. (2006) *Loving the Machine: The Art and Science of Japanese Robots*. Tokyo: Kodansha International.
Houser, K. (2017) Here's everything you need to know about Elon Musk's human/AI brain merge. *Futurism* [Online]. Available at: https://futurism.com/heres-everything-you-need-to-know-about-elon-musks-humanai-brain-merge (Accessed 25 February 2024).
Integral Life. (2006) *Ken Wilber Stops His Brainwaves* [Online]. Available at: https://www.youtube.com/watch?v=LFFMtq5g8N4 (Accessed 20 February 2023).
Jackson, J. C. and Yam, K. C. (2023) The in-credible robot priest and the limits of robot workers. *Scientific American (Opinion)* [Online]. Available at: www.scientificamerican.com/article/the-in-credible-robot-priest-and-the-limits-of-robot-workers/ (Accessed 25 January 2024).
Louv, R. (2005) *Last Child in the Woods: Saving Our Children from Nature Deficit Disorder*. Chapel Hill, NC: Algonquin Books.
Lovelock, J. (2019) *Novacene: The Coming Age of Hyperintelligence*. London: Penguin Books.
Marcus, M. P. (1999) Computer science, the informational and Jewish mysticism. *Technology in Society*, 21, pp. 363–371.
Mim, C. (2010) Why Japanese love robots (And Americans fear them). *MIT Technology Review* [Online]. Available at: www.technologyreview.com/2010/10/12/120635/why-japanese-love-robots-and-americans-fear-them/#:~:text=Given%20that%20Japanese%20culture%20predisposes,hardly%20surprise%20us%20that%20one (Accessed 20 January 2023).
Nuwer, R. (2012) The world's happiest man is a Tibetan monk. *Smithsonian Magazine* [Online]. Available at: www.smithsonianmag.com/smart-news/the-worlds-happiest-man-is-a-tibetan-monk-105980614/ (Accessed 20 February 2024).
Papert, S. (1980) *Mindstorms: Children, Computers and Powerful Ideas*. New York: Basic Books.
Ramirez, D. (Ed.) (2015) *Default Mode Network (DMN): Structural Connectivity, Impairments and Role in Daily Activities*. New York: Nova Science Publishers.
Reiner, P. (2009) Meditation on demand. *Scientific American* [Online]. Available at: www.scientificamerican.com/article/meditation-on-demand/ (Accessed 20 February 2024).
Ricard, M. (2023) *Notebooks of a Wandering Monk*. Cambridge, MA: The MIT Press.
Saxena, A. (2021) *Enlightened Environmentalism: How We Got Here and How to Rescue Our Future*. Irvine: Universal-Publishers.
Seinfeld, J. (2020) *23 Hours to Kill*. Los Gatos, CA: Netflix.
Slade, G. (2009) *Made to Break: Technology and Obsolescence in America*. Cambridge, MA: Harvard University Press.

Slosar, J. R. (2009) *The Culture of Excess: How America Lost Self-Control and Why We Need to Redefine Success*. Westport, CT: Greenwood Publishing.

Southerton, D. (Ed.) (2011) *Encyclopedia of Consumer Culture – Volume 1*. London: Sage.

Stager, G. (2016) Seymour papert (1928–2016). *Nature*, 573, p. 308. [Online]. Available at: www.nature.com/articles/537308a (Accessed 20 March 2023).

Suler, J. R. (2016) *Psychology of the Digital Age: Humans Become Electric*. New York: Cambridge University Press.

Trachtenberg, J. (2004) *Jewish Magic and Superstition*. Philadelphia, PA: University of Pennsylvania Press.

Turkle, S. (2005) *The Second Self: Computers and the Human Spirit*. Cambridge, MA: MIT Press.

7

THE SABBATH AS A TEMPLATE FOR SLOW LIVING

Some of my earliest and happiest memories are of the Friday night *Shabbat* (Sabbath) ceremonies held weekly at our family home. I vividly recall these profoundly Proustian moments with crystalline clarity – the distinctive striking sound and smell of the Cook's matches my mother used to light the Shabbat candles, whose dancing flames of gold and blue illuminated our kitchen table. My father would then recite the *kiddush* the prayer that preceded the Shabbat meal, in ancient Hebrew, taken from the Biblical verse in Genesis. Its slightly archaic-sounding English translation from the *siddur* (prayer book) my father used reads:

> It was evening and it was morning the sixth day. Finished were the heavens and the earth and all the host thereof. And God completed by the seventh day his work which he had made; and he ceased on the seventh day from all his work which he had made. And God blessed the seventh day, and hallowed it; because thereon he ceased from all his work, which God had created for its reproduction.
>
> *(Siddur Avodat Israel 1959, p. 195)*

I recall my grandfather mischievously commentating at the prayer's conclusion – 'see, even God needs a rest!' Despite his humorous intent, there is a deeper teaching implicit in his words – that rest during the Sabbath is Divinely ordained, a sacred time for and place of non-action that theologically constitutes an *imitatio Dei* – an imitation of the Divine.

Following the *brochot* – the blessings, we would drink sweet kiddush wine and eat *challah* – the traditional braided bread of the Sabbath. I particularly

DOI: 10.4324/9781003334972-7

remember savouring the aroma, taste and texture of the large slices of *challah* that had been baked by my grandfather.

My grandfather, Samuel Cohen, was the local baker for the Leeds Jewish community. His shop 'Cohen's Bakery' had originally been founded by his father, Hyman Cohen, in 1898. In addition to being a baker, he was also a Kohein, a member of the traditional priestly caste, descendants of Aaron (the brother of Moses) whose duty remains to bless and teach the Jewish people. I personally believe his way of blessing the people of Leeds was through his baking. The welcoming aroma from his bakery and the dizzying assortment of baked goods – cakes, kitchels, prelatoes and bagels – were as varied as it was mouth-watering. In fact, the only thing he baked which deliberately didn't taste delectable was the *matzah* (unleavened bread) we were expected to eat during the Passover festival. It seems particularly in-keeping with the theme of slow living generally and slow food particularly, that the notoriously dry and tasteless *matzah* is also commonly referred to as the bread of affliction and haste – recollecting the Exodus; the time when the Jewish people were miraculously released from their bondage in Egypt and subsequently commanded to leave the land immediately, without even allowing time for their bread to rise.

Some years later when I was introduced to the *Kabbalah*, Jewish mystical writings, through classes with Professor Daniel Matt, somewhat serendipitously, our very first lesson from the central book of Jewish Mysticism, *Sefer Zohar* (the Book of Splendour) began with a passage related to my Bar Mitzvah portion reading (*Teruma* – offerings made to the priests) and also concerned bread.

In a story, which Professor Matt described as one of the greatest passages in the entire Zohar, a renunciate, hermit-like figure 'who dwelled among the cliffs' (Matt 2009, p. 532), whose simple diet consisted solely of raw wheat kernels, descends into a town and is astounded to discover the vast variety of breads available. He questions the townsfolk as to the ingredients of all these different delicacies and is surprised to learn that each one's primary ingredient is simply wheat. He eventually exclaims, somewhat arrogantly – 'Surely I am king of all of these, since I eat the essence of all these!' (Ibid.).

In other more world-denying, ascetic mystical traditions, this man might have been commended and celebrated for his sturdy devotion to simplicity and renunciation, but in the more sensuous spirituality of the Zohar he appears pitied for his stubborn closed-mindedness, lack of curiosity and consequently self-imposed impoverished palate. The Zohar disapproves of this dismissive mindset, stating:

> Because of that opinion, he knew nothing of the delights of the world, which were lost to him. So it is with one who grasps the principle but is unaware of all those delectable delights deriving, diverging from that principle.
>
> *(Ibid.)*

What at first glance appears to be a simple story about bread becomes an exhortation to explore and discover, particularly in regard to biblical texts – an invitation to hermeneutic inquiry, traversing the revealed literal meaning until one reaches the concealed secret intention. In Hebrew, the term פַּרְדֵּס *Pardes* – Paradise, refers to both an orchard or garden, but also serves as an acronym (PaRDeS) descending into ever deeper depths of meaning and illumination. Beginning with *Pshat* – the literal meaning, progressing to *Remez* – the hint of something beyond, drawing us nearer to *Drash* – which seeks deeper meaning in the moral and allegorical spheres, culminating in *Sod* – the secret inner dimension. When I first began to study the Zohar, I couldn't help but reflect on how my traditional Jewish education had so sorely lacked variety and flavour – subsequently leading me to search and immerse myself in the Eastern traditions of Hinduism, Buddhism and Daoism.

A great deal of my earlier learning at *Cheder* (Jewish Sunday School) had been learning through rote and repetition. We recited the letters of the *Alef Beit*, the Hebrew alphabet, but never learned the histories or mysteries behind the letters. We learned the Jewish law, the *Halakha*, but rarely considered the reasoning or meaning behind the laws – often it was deemed sufficient to know and accept simply that it was a commandment. As an adult, it wasn't a *Halachic* Judaism but rather an *Aggadic* – narrative-centred Judaism, particularly the Hasidic tales of the Baal Shem Tov and Rebbe Nachman that deeply resonated with me. Laws may command and demand our obedience, but lore and stories command our attention, fire our imaginations and fuel our creative capacities. Religion that centres solely on law risks remaining at the literalist level of *pshat*. *Pshat* sees and centres only on what is revealed – it sees only the surface. By contrast, *Sod* gazes deeply, patiently and intently into the depths of what was previously missed or ignored and sees what was previously concealed. In this sense, *pardes* becomes a reminder to take more time in order to look deeper in order to see more, more clearly. This deeper form of seeing is also closely linked to deeper modes of being – described in Hasidic Jewish thought as a psychological shift from *Mochin d'Katnut*'s restricted consciousness to *Mochin d'Gadlut*'s expansive consciousness (Shapiro 2010).

When one looks deeper, even the simple Hebrew letters take on extra dimensions of meaning. Each Hebrew letter also represents a number. Consider the seemingly simple Hebrew letter Pey (see Figure 7.1) as it appears in a Torah scroll – in addition to symbolising the mouth and speech, it is also the number eighty (Haralick 2005).

In the negative space of the letter, hidden in plain sight, is another letter – a *Beit* ב, the second letter of the Hebrew alphabet, and the first letter of the word that both begins the Bible and initiates the whole process of creation – *Bereshit* בְּרֵאשִׁית 'In the beginning . . .'

Kabbalah transformed the fatiguingly familiar into the seductively strange – there were suddenly letters within letters, words within words and worlds within worlds.

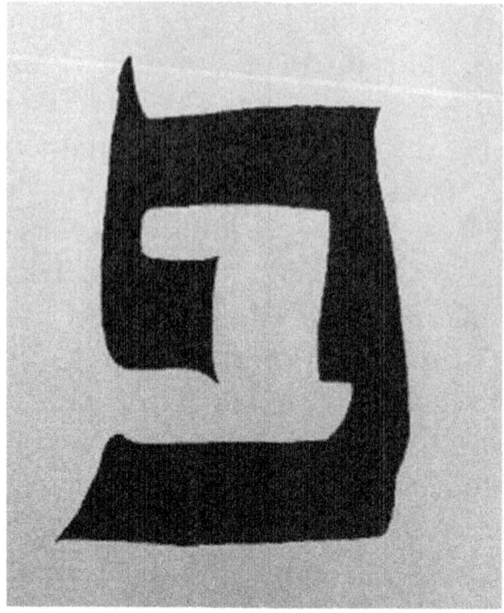

FIGURE 7.1 The letter Pey as it appears in a Torah Scroll – Hand-painted by the calligrapher Zhilu Zhang (author's wife)

The food of the Sabbath likewise has a deeper meaning. Beginning with the sweet kiddush wine. The numerical value of the Hebrew word for secret *Sod* סוֹד is the same as the Hebrew word for wine *Yayin* יַיִן – both are seventy. Hasidic Rabbis are keen to clarify that this is not referring to ordinary intoxication, but rather being drunk on the Divine, in a way that reveals deeper inner secrets.

The traditional two loaves of the bread, the *Challot*, recollect the double portion of heavenly manna that the Jews collected during their sojourn in the desert prior to the dawning of the Sabbath, following their exodus from Egypt. The manna was typically baked into cakes – subsequently, the challah becomes the physical symbol and spiritual descendent of the manna.

As a small curious child, I was amazed at how my grandfather effortlessly plaited the three thick, long strands of dough into the familiar form of the *challah*. Three strands, I later learned, representing the past, present and future, recalling a God who was, who is and will be – braided and baked into unity, offering a taste of timelessness, a foretaste of paradise. The former much-admired Chief Rabbi of the United Kingdom, Sir Jonathan Sacks, eloquently encapsulated this sentiment, in a way that resonates with the Cittaslow Manifesto's reference to 'time reclaimed':

> Shabbat is our moment of eternity in the midst of time. Within the cycle of the week it creates a delicate rhythm of action and reflection, making and enjoying, running and standing still. Without that pause to experience family, community and God, we risk making the journey while missing the view.
>
> *(Sacks 1997, p. 137)*

Erich Fromm, reflecting on Jewish Theology, had reached a similar viewpoint, seeing the Sabbath as akin to psychological liberation, ecological harmony and spiritual realisation:

> The reason why the Sabbath has so central a place within Jewish law lies in the fact that the Sabbath is the expression of the central idea of Judaism: the idea of freedom; the idea of complete harmony between man and nature, man and man; the idea of the anticipation of the messianic time and of man's defeat of time, sadness, and death.
>
> *(Fromm 1966, p. 153)*

The Edenic and Messianic as Both Place and State of Mind

The Hebrew word *Eden* עֵדֶן refers primarily to the qualities of bliss and delight, but also connotes a sense of time and eternity. Eden is synonymous with *pardes* פַּרְדֵּס paradise. The Hebrew word *Pardes* has its etymological roots in the ancient Persian term *Parādaiĵah* referring to an enclosed park or garden. It is also worth emphasising that Eden is the very first *place* to be described in The Bible.

Eden is a primordial place of ease and harmony, where the created is naturally and intimately in tune with the Creator. Popular perceptions of Adam and Eve typically alternate between childish ignorance and childlike innocence. The Kabbalistic view of these first humans is of elevated beings who existed beyond ordinary time and duality, modelled in the image of the Divine – an unprecedented honour which even elicited questioning amongst some of the angelic hosts expressed in Psalms 8:5–6:

> What is frail man that You should remember him, and the son of mortal man that You should be mindful of him?
>
> Yet, You have made him but slightly less than the angels, and crowned him with soul and splendour.
>
> *(Scherman 1996, p. 1443)*

The name given to humankind אָדָם *Adam* has its roots in the Hebrew term for the Earth אֲדָמָה *Adama*. Adam is quite literally 'of the Earth' – an etymological root and timely reminder that may encourage the recognition and cultivation of a more ecological consciousness.

Within Kabbalah, one encounters a fascinating blend of the ecological, theological and psychological in regard to the diagrammatic depiction of *Adam Kadmon* – the primordial man, envisioned as the tree of life. It is only recently that a comprehensive study of these Divinity maps has been carried out by Yossi Chajes (2022) in his encyclopaedic and richly illustrated 'The Kabbalistic Tree'. Chajes painstakingly unveils and explores the arboreal architecture of the cosmos, revealing its sacred symmetries with and correspondences within the human soul.

The tree of life with its ten emanations depicts the creative journey and process – beginning with an unknowable mystical nothingness that extends and expands out into the reality we all see and perceive. From a Kabbalistic perspective, utilising the tree of life, our stream of consciousness may be traced back to a sacred source, enabling one to rediscover the Divine flow or *Shefa* שֶׁפַע, of a river that has its hidden origin in Eden. In Hellner-Eshed's (2009) 'A River Flows from Eden', she conducts a hermeneutical and phenomenological inquiry – emphasising both the exegetical and experiential dimensions of the Zohar. The book appropriately opens with a Zoharic quote that blends the Edenic with the Messianic:

> A river issues from Eden to water the garden (Genesis 2:10) . . . That river flowing forth is called the world that is coming – coming constantly and never ceasing. This is delight of the righteous, to attain this world that is coming, constantly watering the garden and never ceasing.
>
> *(Ibid.)*

Within Jewish cosmology, Eden has become synonymous with Paradise, also called *Olam Haba* – the world to come. It is the place of final rest or *menuchah nechonah* perfect rest, under the wings of the *Shekhinah* – the Divine Presence, in the words of the traditional prayer for the deceased, *El Malei Rachamin* (Compassionate God). But 'world to come' may refer not only to a postmortem destination but also to a future time, a Messianic Age. Despite the contrasting views of who the Messiah will be, what they will do or when they will arrive, the most familiar and oft-quoted verse associated with this age is Isaiah's famous prophetic vision describing the beating of swords into ploughshares – words that still adorn the UN building in New York. The future Messianic world is a world beyond conflict and strife, famously evoked with an image of ecological harmony in Isaiah 11.6 – a time and state of fearlessness that transcends our more familiar pre-redeemed world of predator and prey:

> The wolf will live with the sheep and the leopard will lie down with the kid; and a calf, a lion whelp and a fatling [will walk] together, and a young child will lead them.
>
> *(Scherman 1996, p. 973)*

Both Paradise and Eden have become synonymous with both an ideal outer place and inner psycho-spiritual state of being – a place of harmony, ease and balance. Yet this is not the world we encounter.

This current world, from a Jewish perspective, constitutes a form of Edenic exile, or in Hebrew *Galut* גָּלוּת. In addition to meaning exile, the term *Galut* also conveys a sense of distance from the Divine, captivity and homesickness. The myth of the fall is the biblical narrative that accounts for the origins of our inner and outer disharmonies.

The eating of the forbidden fruit from the tree of the knowledge of good and evil constituted a fall into duality and loss of our primordial unity. In the traditional Biblical narrative, it is God who expels humankind from the Garden of Eden, but in the Zohar, the familiar tale is turned upon its head, and it is suggested that humankind may have been the ones to expel or 'divorce' the Divine (Matt 2004, pp. 297–298).

From a Kabbalistic perspective, the fall represents a constriction of consciousness, a loss of status signified by a sinking into the material realm, seemingly divorced from our former spiritual heights effortlessly attained in the garden. It is also important to note that this is also the mythic origin of all work and human labour, as God rebukes Adam in Genesis 3:19:

> By the sweat of your brow shall you eat bread until you return to the ground from which you are taken: For you are dust, and to dust you shall return.
>
> *(Scherman 1996, p. 9)*

In losing or abandoning the spiritual, we are left only with the material – the dust. It is not the dust we desire to return to; in fact, we fear it as it is synonymous with death – the ultimate terminal division. We yearn for Eden – the tree and source of all life, the perennial place of rest and harmony, where we remember and reconnect with our Divine heritage. As Joni Mitchell memorably sang in her counterculture anthem 'Woodstock', blending contemporary cosmology with biblical theology, singing of our stellar origins and our urgent need to get 'back to the garden' (Mitchell 1970).

The 1960s counterculture's impatience to get 'back to the garden' was perhaps most memorably demonstrated with the proliferation of psychedelics, and the belief that one could circumvent a life of piety and patience, opting instead to simply 'Eat Acid See God'. Theodore Roszak firmly dismissed this spiritual soul hack as a 'counterfeit infinity' (Roszak 1995):

> The gadget-happy American has always been a figure of fun because of his facile assumption that there exists a technological solution to every human problem. It took the great psychedelic crusade to perfect the absurdity by proclaiming that personal salvation and the social revolution can be packed in a capsule.
>
> *(Ibid., p. 177)*

His sentiment would be shared by Abraham Maslow, who at first wondered whether LSD might more easily elicit peak experiences, but soon concluded:

> Even if the drugs were not harmful psychologically, I think they can be harmful spiritually, characterologically, etc. I think it's clearly better to work for your blessings, instead of to buy them. I think an unearned Paradise becomes worthless.
>
> *(Maslow 1966 quoted in Grogan 2013, p. 179)*

The Talmud also contains a cautionary tale for those seeking to storm the gates of heaven – the story of the four great Rabbis who enter the Pardes. Of the four, only one Rabbi, Akiva, 'entered in peace and left in peace' (Koren 2010, p. 261). Of the other three – one died instantly, one lost his mind and one misunderstood what he saw and became a heretic. Some of the darkest chapters of Jewish history often involve tragic tales of those who could not wait for the Messianic Age or the world to come, overcome by the desire to *see* God – despite the clear warning that God gave to Moses in Exodus that 'You will not be able to see My face, for no human can see My face and live' (Scherman 1996, p. 221).

It is significant that we are told that Rabbi Akiva both entered and left in *Shalom* שָׁלוֹם peace – not via the manipulation of mystical formulas or through the purple haze of entheogens. It is the peaceful, settled state of mind that serves as a safe gateway to the Garden of Eden. The prophet Elijah was to experience a similar, subtler revelation when encountering God (recounted in 1 Kings 19:12–13) – the Divine presence was not to be found in the mighty wind, the earthquake or the fire, but rather in the still small voice that followed them.

Tracing the Scent of Eden

Of all the human senses, the one that appears most consistently associated with Eden is the sense of smell. The sweet fragrance of Eden is referred to in many Rabbinic writings, Kabbalistic texts and Hasidic tales. When one thinks of the centre of the Jewish world, one may initially think of Jerusalem – in many ways, Jerusalem becomes the successor to Eden, the site of the first and second temples, constituting an *axis mundi*, a physical manifestation and reflection of a heavenly realm (Chajes 2022); but a lesser known and perhaps equally important site to consider might be the Cave of *Machpelah*, located thirty kilometres south of Jerusalem.

The Hebrew term *Machpelah* מַכְפֵּלָה refers to a doubling or folding, which may refer to its place as the traditional burial site of Adam and Eve, in addition to the Jewish patriarchs and matriarchs – Abraham and Sarah, Isaac and Rebecca, Jacob and Leah. The doubling and folding may also refer to the unusual structural feature of the site, constituting caves within caves. The 'folding' element could refer, even more mysteriously, to the belief that *Machpelah* is a hidden threshold or interdimensional portal between two worlds, the secret, sealed and guarded gateway to Eden (Ginsberg 2023).

In standard *Aggadic* accounts, *Machpelah* was originally discovered when Adam was searching for a burial site for Eve, following the mythic fall and resulting Edenic exile. Upon discovering the cave, he was drawn to a familiar homely fragrance, the sweet nostalgic scent of Eden, at which point he is informed by Divine decree that he must venture no further. Both the Bible and Zohar similarly recount Abraham expending particular effort to contractually secure the site as a future family burial plot, as he recognised the spiritual significance of the location, as it emitted divine lights and sweet scents discernible only to him.

There remained a belief that the Edenic aroma, in addition to being a portent of the future messianic age, still accompanies and emanates from the righteous in the world, and from righteous acts. In Zevin's (1992) treasury of Hasidic tales on the Torah, he includes several stories pertaining to the 'flavour' and even the 'whiff' (Ibid., pp. 104–107) of Eden. In these stories, it is not only the *Tzadikim* (the saintly and righteous) that may emit the Edenic scent, it may also arise due to acts of ordinary faith and loving-kindness. One such story involves an impoverished woman with a bare kitchen, desperately preparing a meal for her husband's honoured guest, the great Rabbi David of Lelov. Due to her faith and loving preparation of a very simple meal, Rabbi David later remarked to his wife, 'When I was at my friend's house in the village, I ate some kind of delicacy, and in it I really tasted the flavour of the garden of Eden' (Ibid., p. 104).

One particularly curious Hasidic tale relates to one of the early founding figures of Hasidism, Rabbi Menachem Mendel of Vitebsk (1730–1788 CE), and his reputed ability to detect the coming of the Messiah through scent alone. The story concerns the prematurely exuberant disciples of the Rabbi, who rushed into his house exclaiming that they had heard a heavenly proclamation, the blowing of the *shofar* (the Ram's horn), and excitedly informed their teacher that the Messiah's arrival was imminent. The Rabbi calmly proceeded to the nearest window and upon opening it, stuck his head outside to sniff the air outside – only to announce, much to the disappointment of his students, that the Messiah was not yet here. The explanation as to why the Rabbi needed to sniff the air outside is that due to the holiness of the Rabbi and his home as a sacred place for the study of Torah, the air within his home was already suffused with the redolence of redemption.

Getting Back to the Garden

Through an Analytical Psychological frame, Eden may be seen as a mythic motif, a primordial place and an archetypal setting. As such, variants of the garden paradise, trees of life and sacred rivers are found throughout the world's wisdom traditions and mythologies.

For Jung, Eden evokes the mandalas of Hinduism and Buddhism (Jung 1990, p. 35), which are themselves intended as imaginal maps for psycho-spiritual integration, which constitutes the Analytical Psychologist's goal of individuation – becoming more fully Self-realised. In traditional Tibetan iconography and Jungian Psychology, the mandala becomes a transformative meeting point between one's physical place and one's state of mind:

> The outer world, one's body and state of mind, and the totality can all be seen as mandala. The constructed form of a mandala has as its basic structure a palace with a centre and four gates in the cardinal directions.
>
> *(Baker 2012, p. 215)*

Traditional depictions of Eden also display a quaternity – with the tree of life located at the centre, the river flowing from Eden divides and diverges into four rivers which flow in four directions. This mandalic layout is found in many other mythic realms. A great many traditions also tell of hidden or lost lands that only the spiritually realised can discover – Arcadia, Agartha, Atlantis, Avalon, Buyan, Kitezh, Kunlun, Penglai, Tír na nÓg, etc.

Of particular note is the hidden realm of *Shambhala* in Tibetan Buddhism, or the concealed land of *Olmo Lungring* in the pre-Buddhist Tibetan Bön, which also possesses four rivers that flow in four directions. Some scholars even contend that the word *Olmo* may be a Semitic loanword related to the Hebrew term *Olam* עוֹלָם which translates as world, space, time and eternity, which is in turn related to the verb *Alam* עָלַם which means to conceal (Martin 2007, pp. 104–105). Another element these places share is their ontological ambiguity, with many questioning whether they are physical places or spiritual realms – the most common answers tend to take a middle way.

A closely related concept is that of the *beyul* སྦས་ཡུལ or hidden valleys of Tibetan Buddhism. In Ian Baker's (2004) definitive book on *beyul*, the Dalai Lama provides the following description in his introduction:

> Centuries ago, texts were discovered in Tibet describing beyul, hidden-lands where the essence of the Buddhist Tantras is said to be preserved for future generations.
>
> . . . When approached with an awareness of the emptiness and luminosity underlying all appearances, they can encourage us to expand our vision not only of ourselves, but of reality itself.
>
> *(Dalai Lama quoted in Baker 2004, pp. 1–2)*

Returning once more to the theme of a more expansive consciousness and vision, one may consider the Tibetan term *daknang* དག་སྣང་ – pure vision. In a similar vein to Abraham's prophetic vision which enabled him to see the hidden lights of Eden, so too must one possess an awakened mind in order to perceive the *beyul* – even then one may not always enter. In the Bible, it takes a particular prophet, Moses, to find the promised land; in Tibetan Buddhism, it takes a special individual known as a *tertön* གཏེར་སྟོན – a revealer of treasures, to locate and ultimately unlock the *beyul* allowing others to enter.

The unlocked *beyul* that Baker explores is the land of Pemako, which straddles the borders of both China and India, and remains a popular, though difficult to access, Buddhist pilgrimage site. *Beyuls* are considered particularly powerful places for spiritual practice. One especially enthusiastic visitor to Pemako was the French Buddhist monk Mattieu Ricard who fondly recounted:

> It was the very picture of the image of the mythical Shangri-La, the paradise of James Hilton's novel Lost Horizon, later adapted for film by Frank Capra. A place set apart from the world, where everything feels simple, peaceful and harmonious, and where there is nothing to do but no one seems to feel the slightest need to keep busy. A place replete with blessings unchanged from time immemorial, where every atom of earth, water, and air seems to quiver with the presence of timeless wisdom and compassion.
>
> *(Ricard 2023, p. 652)*

Hilton's Shangri-La appears in so many ways to be a synthesis between Eden and Shambhala – a paradisical garden hidden somewhere in the Himalayas. In popular culture, Hilton's 'Lost Horizon' appeared to recover and revitalise deeply held utopian yearnings for a world still reeling from the cataclysmic horrors of the First World War. The book was originally published in 1933, the same year the Reichstag burned, and the Nazis rose to power in Germany. The feature film that followed was released in 1937, when the Second World War had already begun in Asia, with Japan's invasion of China. In Capra's filmed version, Shangri-La's High Lama explains the place's purpose to the tale's complex protagonist Hugh Conway, in a manner that emphasises the importance of spiritual conservation and the preservation of cultural memory:

> It is the entire meaning and purpose of Shangri-La. It came to me in a vision long, long ago. I saw all the nations strengthening, not in wisdom, but in the vulgar passions and the will to destroy. I saw their machine power multiplying until a single weaponed man might match a whole army. I foresaw a time when man exalting in the technique of murder, would rage so hotly over the world, that every book, every treasure would be doomed to destruction. This vision was so vivid and so moving that I determined to gather together all things of beauty and culture that I could and preserve them here against the doom toward which the world is rushing.
>
> *(Lost Horizon 1937)*

Of Gardens and Gardening

In Simon Schama's (1993) 'Landscape and Memory', both the individual and collective mythologies of the natural world are explored. Schama begins with his own early recollections of his Jewish upbringing, including the festival of Tu BiShvat – the Jewish New Year for trees:

> So we recited the blessings over our paper tree as the sprouted descendent of the Tree of Life, guarded in Eden, so the Scripture said, by an angel with a flaming sword. Our sixpenny-worth of arboriculture was re-creating that garden in a new Zion. And if a child's vision of nature can already be loaded with complicating memories, myths and meanings, how much more elaborately wrought it the frame through which our adult eyes survey the landscape.
>
> *(Ibid., p. 6)*

For Schama, the landscape cannot be meaningfully separated from the mind – we internalise our natural world and in doing so we may often idealise it. Schama does not succumb to romantic idealisations of the landscape however, poetically capturing the ambivalence of the natural world through his consideration of 'Arcadia Redesigned' (Ibid., p. 517):

> There have always been two kinds of arcadia: shaggy and smooth; dark and light; a place of bucolic leisure and a place of primitive panic.
>
> *(Ibid.)*

One might note that the myth of the biblical fall both precedes and leads to this duality. In fact, it is precisely the Edenic exile that transforms the world of bucolic leisure into one of panic, but the original primordial state is far from primitive, but rather a state of expansive ease and delight.

The physical garden has traditionally been a place of idealised natural order, but more recently there has been a tendency to recover and embrace the natural state. When gardening one might reflectively inquire as to whether one is seeking to impose order or recover a natural order?

The psychological benefits of gardening are well-documented and manifold, with research demonstrating improvements in 'emotional, social, vocational, physical and spiritual domains' (Clatworthy et al. 2013, p. 214). Gardening may be a form of psychotherapy in the more etymological sense of the word, meaning mind/soul healing. Even one of the more materialist-minded, founding fathers of the scientific method, Francis Bacon (1561–1626), recognised that there was something spiritually elevating in the act of gardening:

> God Almighty first planted a garden, and indeed, it is the purest of human pleasures; it is the greatest refreshment to the spirits of man; without which buildings and palaces are but gross handiworks; and a man shall ever see,

> that when ages grow to civility and elegancy, men come to build stately, sooner than to garden finely; as if gardening were the greater perfection.
> *(Bacon quoted in Montagu 1859, p. 51)*

At the time Bacon was writing, the most familiar form of garden remained the Italianate garden (Hunt 1999); which had its roots in renaissance ideals, reflecting age-old aspirations to master the natural world. The Italian style emphasised custodianship, an imposed order which found expression through regimental rows of trees, lines of tightly clipped, painstakingly maintained topiaries and flower beds laid in rather rigid geometric grids.

A century or so later, Lancelot 'Capability' Brown (1716–1783) would pioneer a more naturalistic approach to gardening and landscaping. His nickname 'capability' was said to be the result of his being able to not only perceive but cultivate, reveal and realise the aesthetic potential of the many stately grounds he designed (Phibbs 2017), including Harewood House in Leeds, where we would often visit as a family. When wandering through these gardens, it is often easy to forget that they are the result of a great deal of human labour and planning, that what we see is an often masterful imitation of nature rather than nature herself. This imitation of nature can also be seen in some of the most famous gardens of China and Japan.

The rock gardens of Suzhou in China deliberately emulate and recreate in miniature, mountainous landscapes through the placing large *Taihu* stones in order to create captivating centrepieces (Keswick 2003). *Taihu* stones, named after the local *Taihu* lake, consist of curiously shaped limestone that has been naturally carved and smoothed through millennia of erosion. These stones become inspiring examples of the effortless artistry of nature, the original found art of Daoism.

Likewise, the classic Japanese Zen Gardens of Kyoto replicate the natural world in a way that intentionally reflects and elicits a more meditative and creative state of mind. It is common to see the Zen Garden primarily as a contemplative tool and object of focus – its inherent harmony and creative use of space are intended to recover and resonate with our own inner equanimity and appreciation of emptiness. There is however an equally important aesthetic element of imagination and creativity, embedded within their construction. The Japanese term *mitate-e* 見立絵 expresses this more playful way of seeing and experiencing the garden (Nguyen 2018). *Mitate-e* may transform the character-filled, craggy stones into leaning or sitting Buddhas and Bodhisattvas, the deep green beds of star moss become lush forests, and the carefully raked gravel, concentric, circular or waved into the waves of the world's oceans or the ripples upon the surface of a pond after a pebble has been dropped in. In the Japanese garden, nature has undergone a distillation and miniaturisation, not with the intention of mere imitation but also of refining. This philosophy and process is encapsulated in the lifelong pruning, tying and bending of the branches of a bonsai tree. This deliberate stunting and constant manicuring of tiny trees may seem entirely at odds with another central Japanese principle of *wabi-sabi* 侘び寂び (Koren 2008) the profound appreciation of the natural state, unadorned, non-contrived; typically prizing objects and features which appear weathered, worn and rustic – but this apparent paradox doesn't appear to disturb the Japanese psyche.

More contemporary trends in gardening and landscaping appear to be adopting a much more *wabi-sabi* aesthetic and *wu wei* sentiment. In 2021, the Chelsea Flower Show awarded a gold award to Peter Chmiel and Chin Chen's Guangzhou Garden – a harmonious confluence of latticed wooden structures, plants and a central stream fed by a concealed waterfall. The garden's description restates some core principles of biophilic design:

> The garden highlights the benefits of responsible city planning and how planners must work in harmony with nature to better connect people with the natural world.
>
> *(Royal Horticultural Society 2021)*

In 2022, the Gold Winners were Urquhart and Hunt's Landscape Design titled 'A Rewilding Britain Landscape', which gave the appearance of a restored wilderness as opposed to a more traditional and manicured garden:

> For us it's about letting go of the constructs of what a garden should be. As part of that deconstruction, we're really excited to bring in a natural landscape rather than a garden.
>
> *(Urquhart quoted in Royal Horticultural Society 2022)*

Increasingly, it appears that we may be learning to accept and integrate the shadow, the perceived wildness of the wilderness, replacing primitive panic with an attitude of acceptance and a sense of belonging.

Slow Living – A Recipe for Recovery

During the global pandemic, I recall the joy and wonder expressed by some of my Nepalese friends as they began to share photos of a pristine and majestic Mount Everest on social media. This was the first time in their collective memory that the sacred mountain, which locals know as *Sagarmatha* – Goddess of the Sky, had become clearly visible from Kathmandu. The small nation of Nepal lies between India and China – a popular tourist destination, known for its busy, bustling, often overcrowded, frequently frenetic streets and neighbourhoods. A nationwide lockdown, beginning in March 2020, and the subsequent halting of activity in factories and construction sites, and the lack of cars, lorries and planes had led to a rather dramatic and visible improvement in the air quality, which had previously been determined as constituting an environmental and public health risk by the World Health Organisation – potentially even more harmful than the Covid-19 virus. During lockdown, somewhat ironically, many inhabitants of the Kathmandu Valley suddenly discovered that they could breathe easier and deeper, see clearer and farther, than ever before. It was as if the valley had revealed or restored itself back into a *beyul*, a paradise on Earth.

Closer to home, many appeared to be using the lockdown to discover new hobbies. The sheer scale of people engaging in gardening and baking led to a profusion of online articles all seeking to understand the psychology underlying these behaviours, for example, 'Why We're All Gardening and Baking So Much – How self-determination theory can help you survive the long, drawn-out pandemic?' (Stuhlberg 2020). These articles all typically emphasised the role of regaining a sense of control, mastery and self-efficacy during challenging times of uncertainty. At the same time, the Royal College of Psychiatrists was offering a free webinar promoting Stuart-Smith's (2020) 'The Well-Gardened Mind', which explored familiar themes of biophilia, the healing, stress-reducing and restorative effects of natural environments. Yet I would argue that there is a larger lesson still to learn through the activities of gardening and baking. Both activities impart the importance of learning to slow down and synchronise ourselves with a more natural, harmonious and humanising pace; ultimately letting go of the seductive illusion of and obsessive need for control.

Kneading ever faster or repeatedly raising the temperature of the oven ever higher does not make the bread any better. Popping the young green buds prematurely won't help the flowers to bloom any earlier or more beautifully. The secret to great baking as with gardening are the self-same qualities of slow living – attentiveness and patience that lead to letting be, trusting the process, and allowing nature to take its course. This is the *wu wei* of the Daoists – the realisation that through letting be we allow ourselves time and space to authentically become.

Slow living is the antidote to that deadening, desensitising automaticity that can so subtly and insidiously come to dominate so many of our daily routines, consequently leading to a dulling of the palate of daily life:

> The quest for slowness, which begins as a simple rebellion against the impoverishment of taste in our lives, makes it possible to rediscover taste.
> *(Petrini quoted in Shultz 2012, p. 234)*

This rediscovery ultimately lies in the recovery of novelty – hence my repeated references to Eden. Eden is the beginning of beginnings, the first of all things. This Edenic consciousness finds a cross-cultural counterpart in the *sho shin* 初心 beginner's mind (Suzuki 2020) of Zen Buddhism, which approaches the world with a fresh, childlike openness and curiosity.

And so, in conclusion, I return to my cherished childhood memory, my family and I gathered around the kitchen table on Shabbat. It is pertinent that with the destruction of the Jewish temple during the sacking of Jerusalem, millennia ago, the Rabbis made the decision to move the sacred centre of Jewish life to the kitchen table (Harper 2023). One may even begin to identify an imaginal lineage beginning in the Garden of Eden, moving to the Temple of Jerusalem, and finally being transferred to the humble kitchen table of the family home – the table symbolically transforming into a tabernacle. Both the Sabbath and slow living seek to cultivate that simultaneously creative and playful way of seeing and being that transforms ordinary perception into poetic vision.

Slow living offers us a way back to a golden age, the stillness and truth of the *Satya Yuga*, in the chaotic midst of the Kali Yuga. It is the *citta* slowing of the Buddha's Dharma – the decelerated heart and mind that sees clearly and subsequently acts compassionately. It is the Edenic encounter offering a much-needed Sabbath for the world. A time to power down our machines and return to the garden.

In living more slowly, more mindfully and intentionally, with patience and through practice, we gradually relearn to discern that still small voice that calls us home.

References

Baker, I. (2004) *The Heart of the World: Journey to the Last Secret Place*. New York: Penguin Press.

Baker, I. (2012) *The Dalai Lama's Secret Temple*. New York: Thames and Hudson.

Chajes, J. H. (2022) *The Kabbalistic Tree*. Philadelphia, PA: The Pennsylvania State University Press.

Clatworthy, J., Hinds, J. and Camic, P. (2013) Gardening as a mental health intervention: A review. *Mental Health Review*, 18(4), pp. 214–225.

Fromm, E. (1966) *You Shall Be as Gods: A Radical Reinterpretation of the Old Testament and Its Tradition*. New York: Fawcett Premier.

Ginsberg, L. (2023) *Legends of the Jews (Vol. 1–4): Bible Times and Characters from the Creation to Esther*. Glasgow: Good Press.

Grogan, J. (2013) *Encountering America: Humanistic Psychology, Sixties Culture & the Shaping of the Modern Self*. New York: Harper Collins Publishers.

Haralick, R. (2005) *The Inner Meaning of the Hebrew Letters*. Lanham, MD: Rowman and Littlefield Publishers.

Harper, V. M. (2023) *Loaves of Torah: Exploring the Jewish Year Through Challah*. New York: Reform Jewish Publishing.

Hellner-Eshed, M. (2009) *A River Flows from Eden: The Language of Mystical Experience in the Zohar*. Stanford, CA: Stanford University Press.

Hunt, J. (Ed.) (1999) *The Italian Garden: Art, Design and Culture*. Cambridge: Cambridge University Press.

Jung, C. G. (1990) *The Archetypes and the Collective Unconscious*. Princeton, NJ: Princeton University Press.

Keswick, M. (2003) *The Chinese Garden: History, Art and Architecture*. Cambridge, MA: Harvard University Press.

Koren, I. (2010) *The Mystery of the Earth: Mysticism and Hasidism in the Thought of Martin Buber*. Leiden: Brill.

Koren, L. (2008) *Wabi-Sabi for Artists, Designers, Poets and Philosophers*. Inverness, CA: Imperfect Publishing.
Lost Horizon (1937) Directed by Frank Capra. Los Angeles: Columbia Pictures.
Marcus, M. P. (1999) Computer science, the informational and Jewish mysticism. *Technology in Society*, 21, pp. 363–371.
Martin, D. (2007) Olmo lungring – A holy place here and beyond. In: Karmay, S. G. and Watt, J. (Eds.) *Bon: The Magic Word: The Indigenous Religion of Tibet*. London: Philip Wilson Publishers, pp. 99–123.
Matt, D. (2004) *The Zohar: Pritzker Edition* (Volume I). Stanford, CA: Stanford University Press.
Matt, D. (2009) *The Zohar: Pritzker Edition* (Volume V). Stanford, CA: Stanford University Press
Mitchell, J. (1970) *Woodstock*. New York: Reprise Records.
Montagu, B. (1859) *The Works of Francis Bacon Lord Chancellor of England: With a Life of the Author: Volume I*. Philadelphia, PA: Parry and McMillan.
Nguyen, A. (2018) *New Essays in Japanese Aesthetics*. Lanham, MD: Lexington Books.
Phibbs, J. (2017) *Place-Making: The Art of Capability Brown*. Swindon: Historic England.
Ricard, M. (2023) *Notebooks of a Wandering Monk*. Cambridge, MA: The MIT Press.
Roszak, T. (1995) *The Making of a Counter Culture*. Berkeley, CA: University of California Press.
Royal Horticultural Society (2021) Guangzhou China: Guangzhou garden [Online]. Available at: www.rhs.org.uk/shows-events/rhs-chelsea-flower-show/Gardens/2021/guangzhou-china-guangzhou-garden (Accessed 15 March 2024).
Royal Horticultural Society (2022) Meet the designers: Rewilding Britain [Online]. Available at: www.rhs.org.uk/shows-events/rhs-chelsea-flower-show/news/2022/rewilding-garden#:~:text=At%20the%20RHS%20Chelsea%20Flower,%2Dyear%20absence%3A%20the%20beaver (Accessed 15 March 2024).
Sacks, J. (1997) *Faith in the Future: The Ecology of Hope and the Restoration of Family Community and Faith*. Macon, GA: Mercer University Press.
Schama, S. (1993) *Landscape and Memory*. London: Fontana Press.
Scherman, N. (Ed.) (1996) *The Stone Edition Tanach: The Torah/Prophets/Writings: The Twenty-Four Books of the Bible Newly Translated and Annotated*. New York: Mesorah Publications.
Shapiro, R. (2010) *Tanya the Masterpiece of Hasidic Wisdom: Selections Annotated and Explained*. Nashville: Turner Publishing Company.
Shultz, K. (2012) On establishing a more authentic relationship with food: From Heidegger to Oprah on slowing down fast food. In: Frye, J. and Bruner, M. (Eds.) *The Rhetoric of Food: Discourse, Materiality and Power*. New York: Routledge, pp. 222–237.
Siddur Avodat Yisrael. (1959) Tel Aviv: Sinai Publishing.
Stuart-Smith, S. (2020) *The Well-Gardened Mind: Rediscovering Nature in the Modern World*. New York: Scribner.
Stuhlberg, B. (2020) Why we're all gardening and baking so much – how self-determination theory can help you survive the long, drawn-out pandemic. *Outside Magazine* [Online]. Available at: www.outsideonline.com/health/wellness/why-gardening-baking-popular-during-pandemic/ (Accessed 23 January 2023).
Suzuki, S. (2020) *Zen Mind, Beginner's Mind: Informal Talks on Zen Meditation and Practice*. Boulder, CO: Shambhala Publications.
Zevin, S. Y. (1992) *A Treasury of Chassidic Tales on the Torah*. New York: Mesorah Publications.

INDEX

Note: *Page numbers in italic indicate a figure on the corresponding page.*

Printed in Great Britain
by Amazon

56172301R00084